AF208591

Copyright Notice

Disclaimer

The information provided in this book is based upon my
interpretations of the research available and upon my
experiences and is for educational purposes only. I am
not a doctor, and, therefore, you should have a dialogue
with your physician before you enter this program to
insure if the advices in this program are appropriate for
your individual circumstances. The information in this
book is meant for people with a BMI over 25+ and for
healthy people only.

If you have any health issues or pre-existing conditions,
please have a dialogue with your physician before you
follow this program. If your physician tells you that this

program is good for you but you start to feel dizzy during the program, please contact your physician immediately.

The author is not responsible for any damages, liabilities, injuries, perceived or real from using this product.

About the author

My name is Pontus Olsson and I am 24 years old and I come from the Nordic country Sweden. I have always been interested in sports, healthy eating and helping people. It all started at the age of six years old where I started to play football for five years. Then I moved on to another sport, which was free athletics, where my interest for running started to grow. I started to compete in the distance of 800 m where my personal record is 2:10 minutes. I was training free athletics for five years and then I decided to work out on my own, so I started to run all distances from 5 km to 42,2 km. I combined the running with strength training which I am still doing. My training goals for the year 2018 are to run a half marathon (21,1 km) under 1:20 hours, a marathon (42,2 km) under 3:05 hours and become stronger at the gym and stay as healthy as possible.

My personal records in running are: 800 m (2:10 minutes), 5K (18:15 minutes), 10K (38:51 minutes), half marathon (1:23:57 hours, 30K (2:07:00 hours) and marathon (3:10:08) hours. The marathon, I have only run twice in my lifetime so far.

When I was in the age of 14 years old, I wrote a very short book about healthy food for weight loss. I didn't sell it, I was just very interesting in healthy foods. When I turned 15 years old, I started to study society with a focus on sport at high school. During this period of studying my interest of training, health and nutrition started to grow like crazy. When I decided to study at college, I knew exactly what I wanted to do, I wanted to study about health, training, nutrition and how the body works. So, I applied for an education called Health Science with a focus on Biomedical Sciences, this gave me, when I was 22 years old a Degree of Bachelor of Science in Biomedical Sciences (180 credits). During this education, I also wrote an Examination Project Work in Health Science with the title "Is the human being affected in different ways by endurance training on fasting or non-fasting stomach in terms of physiological markers in the body?", I passed with Distinction at that Project.

Förlag: BoD – Books on Demand, Stockholm, Sverige

Tryck: BoD – Books on Demand, Norderstedt, Tyskland

ISBN: 978-91-7785-561-3

Table of contents

INTERMITTENT FASTING FOR A HEALTHY LIFESTYLE WEIGHT LOSS AND FAT BURNING PROGRAM

BY

PONTUS OLSSON

Chapter 1

What does intermittent fasting mean?

Intermittent fasting is a lifestyle where you fast (avoid some sort of food, not water, tea or coffee) for 16 – 20 hours and then feed (consume food) for 4 – 8 hours during a day. The intermittent fasting lifestyle is based upon the hours of the day. If you, for example, start your feeding window (the time of the day where you can eat all the food during a day) at 12 am then you need to consume all your energy from the food before 8 pm. No one will control you when you will start the fast and stop the fast, the only person that decides when you can consume food and fast is you! You are your own boss of your lifestyle and so of your diet. This is the best thing about intermittent fasting – you can eat whenever you want to. Personally, I vary my feeding and fasting windows for almost each day. Some days I can start my feeding window at 2 pm and stop the feeding window between 6 pm and 8 pm, it depends on when I want to eat and what I have planned that day. You should choose your feeding window so it fits with your work, school and/or free time.

Intermittent fasting does not mean that you should eat every 2 – 3 hours during a day. When you follow this lifestyle, you should aim for eating 1 – 3 meals a day depending on how much food you can eat in a sitting and what you have planned during the day. I usually eat 2 meals per day and sometimes just one. The most important thing about intermittent fasting is that you push your first meal until you have fasted for 16 – 20 hours because there is where the magic happens. All the health benefits from intermittent fasting comes in when you fast for more than 16 hours each day. You can read about the health benefits in chapter 7.

When a person talks about fasting many people associate this with starvation which is the total opposite of fasting. Starvation is a state where the body does not get enough of food for a long time which can lead to a deteriorated metabolic state and even death. When a person starves, it is not on purpose, it is because he or she cannot find food and this leads to a deterioration of health and the lack of nutrients (1).

Chapter 2

For how long time should you utilize intermittent fasting?

A lot of people fast every 2 – 3 day a week, some people fast 1 day a week and other people fast every day. Personally, I fast every day for 16 – 20 hours. I have realized that the longer the fast is the more body fat and weight I lose. The research also agrees with this fact. I never eat when I wake up because when you eat, your fat burning process inhibits and you cannot lose fat and weight until the insulin (a peptide hormone which is secreted through increased levels of glucose in the blood and functions as a regulator of the blood sugar levels in the body) from the food has lowered in your body. During the fasting window, you increase your fat burning process so that the body must get rid of fat to get energy.

By this, I mean you should fast every day for 16 – 20 hours to get the maximum effect from the intermittent fasting lifestyle. You should also fast until you have reached the bodyweight that you want to have, this can take weeks to months to years depending on your current body fat percentage and bodyweight. When you have reached your weight that you are happy with, then you should increase your calories so you always eat in maintenance (the state where you eat the same calories as your body expends) (2). In one study, where the participants were overweight and obese, they lost 3 – 8 % of their bodyweight by fasting each other day for 2 – 24 weeks (3). I think that the participants would have lost that amount of bodyweight faster if they fasted every day.

Chapter 3

Disadvantages/health risks with intermittent fasting

If you are on a diet, where you are in a calorie deficit (you eat less than your body expends in a day) for too long, then bulimia can emerge. Bulimia is an eating disorder where you consume all the food very fast and in a very short period of time (less than two hours). Bulimia is also associated with loss of control which means that you cannot stop consume food. When you have consumed the food then you try to vomit or use laxatives just to get rid of the food. Bulimia can lead to depression, anxiety, wounds in the mouth, diarrhea, blood vomiting, heart-rhythm disturbances, wounds on your hands, swollen spotting glands, dental injuries, edema, swelling and reflux concerns (4). Bulimia can lead to a lot of issues if you do not search for treatment (5). However, there is no clinical trials that have shown that intermittent fasting can cause eating disorders (3).

Another disadvantage with intermittent fasting is if you eat all the calories in four hours in a day (20 hours long fast) (2). This can lead to that you won't be able to consume all the calories that you are supposed to consume in a day just because of the big amount of food. If you do not consume the number of calories you are supposed to in a day, it can lead to the lack of some vitamins and minerals that are vital for you.

The protein in the body can break down during short periods of fasting, this is called proteolysis. The research has analyzed this process during a night fast (where you fast from the evening until the breakfast next morning) and 60 hours after the last meal which means that it is not sure if the proteolysis increases by fasting 16 – 20 hours a day. One study showed that urea and muscle proteolysis did not increase after a 36 hour long fast but it increased after a 60 hour long fast. Earlier studies of fasting show that the breakdown of protein starts after three days of fasting (72 hour long fast) (2) and this type of fasting is very difficult to stick to and it is not what this program is designed for. I would not fast that long! When you fast longer than a night fast the body starts to break down glycogen and fat. The resting metabolism increases after a short period of fasting but is most effective after 36 – 48 hours of fasting (2).

If a person consumes very little calories in a day by eating low calorie diets or by semistarvation, it can lead to hyperphagia (you do not feel satiated and keep on eating too much calories which lead to overweight and obesity) and higher levels of fat mass (total body fat) than you had when you started the diet/lifestyle. Less than 800 calories a day is way too little and this can cause, as I wrote before, the lack of some vitamins and minerals and even protein, carbohydrates and fats that are vital for you. A lot of people think that if they eat very low calories (less than 1000 calories or even 800 calories a day) they will lose weight like crazy and their overweight and obesity will be gone forever... This is not true! In fact, this is the opposite of what the research shows. If you eat 800 calories a day or 1600 – 2000 calories a day the result of the weight loss will almost be the same, but it is way healthier to consume more calories because then you can easily consume all the vitamins, minerals and macronutrients (protein, carbohydrates and fats) that you need in a day which are also important for the weight loss. If you eat too little calories, like 800 – 1000 calories a day for a long period of time, your body will trigger biological adjustments that will help you if you want to gain weight with more fat mass in percentage (2). When you eat too little calories, your body must counteract glucose deficiency which mainly occurs through increased muscle protein degradation. This means that when you eat more calories the next time, you will have less muscle mass and more fat mass. Proteins can be converted into sugar but fat cannot be converted into sugar and that is why we get more fat mass after eating too little calories for a while. After a while of low calorie intake, the body starts to produce ketone bodies which lead to increased fat oxidation. But eating too little calories for a long time is not recommended (6).

Chapter 4

What causes obesity and weight gain?

Diet-induced obesity and lack of the hormone leptin (is produced by the white fat cells and is secreted a lot more if the person has more body fat) is associated with bigger sized meals which causes weight gain. The number of calories you consume in a day does not only depend on the meal's size but on the total amount of meals you consume in a day and the connection between the amount of meals and the size of the meal are affected by peptides like CCK (cholecystokinin), amylin and GLP-1 (glucagon-like peptide-1) (3). When you use intermittent fasting to lose weight, noradrenaline (can also be called norepinephrine is a stress hormone which makes us happy and has many functions related to stressful situations) in the medial hypothalamus and the peptide NPY (neuropeptide Y) in the hypothalamus arcuate nucleus increase which can affect the meal pattern of your diet. This is only one factor among many which shows that intermittent fasting, smaller sizes of the meals and changed meal patterns can have positive results on these dietary patterns (3).

The most common example, and the truth, about what causes obesity is that the calories a person consumes in a day are higher than the calories the body expends in a day. This leads to increased fat in the fatty tissues (7). If you eat more calories than your body expends in a day, your fat cells will produce more fat in the fatty tissues which is not the goal we aim for.

In one study, the authors discussed that the fat rich meals the most people consume in their diets are a factor which leads to obesity among humans (8).

Chapter 5

What are the consequences of obesity?

Obese and overweight individuals have a higher risk of developing diabetes type II and cancer such as colon cancer, breast cancer, prostate cancer and liver cancer (9).

Obesity can also cause problems such as hyperinsulinemia (too high levels of insulin in the blood), hyperleptinemia (too high levels of leptins in the blood), hyperglycemia (too high levels of glucose in the blood – high blood sugar), insulin resistance (the cells in the body do not respond effectively to insulin) and even glucose intolerance (higher levels of glucose in the blood) (8). Other problems that can occur by being obese are non-alcoholic fatty liver disease (one form of fatty liver, a liver disorder), cardiovascular diseases (diseases that affect blood vessels or the heart), hyperlipidemia (higher levels of some or all lipoproteins or lipids in the blood) and hypertension (high blood pressure). These last three mentioned problems are called the metabolic syndrome (10). A big trouble that comes with obesity is decreased adiponectin (a protein hormone that regulates the levels of glucose and the breakdown of fatty acids) and increased leptin synthesis which is thought to be a step in the direction of developing cancer through effects on inflammation, insulin sensitivity (how sensitive the body is to insulin – higher insulin sensitivity requires less insulin to be secreted which is healthier than low insulin sensitivity), apoptosis (programmed cell death) and cell proliferation (increased number of cells) (11).

The mood is highly affected by gaining weight and being obese / overweight. In a study, it was showed that people who gain weight or already are overweight / obese tend to be more depressed than normal weighted people and even people on a weight loss diet (12).

Chapter 6

How to treat obesity?

If you want to treat your obesity and get leaner and smaller then you must reduce the calories you eat in a day so you eat under maintenance and increase the physical activity which means that your body expends more calories in a day and this allows you to eat more calories in a day and still be under the maintenance level (7). Well… How do you know what your maintenance level is? I will teach you this in chapter 20.

If you have a hard time losing weight because you cannot reduce the calorie intake then mindfulness is a great tool to help you with the weight loss. This tool may help you with the diet, your social network, your self-confidence, your training and much more, according to a study made on women and weight loss (12). Another tool that may help you with the weight loss is called "modelling" which means that you watch how other people behave in situations that you fear or have trouble with (the weight loss, for example) and then retrain and modify physiological conditions like "I can't lose weight because I like food way too much" into something positive like "I have to reduce the calorie intake to be as healthy as possible and live the life I want to live" (12).

Chapter 7

Health benefits of intermittent fasting

Intermittent fasting is a very healthy and effective lifestyle that is known for its health benefits. Intermittent fasting (a fast for 16 – 20 hours in a day) combined with physical activity can reduce the risk for obesity-related diseases (7). The physiological factors that lead to lower risk for obesity-related diseases are improved body composition (increased muscle mass percentage and reduced body fat percentage) (7).

Another health benefit of intermittent fasting (a fast for 24 hours) is that glucose- and lipid metabolism decreases. Within the first 24 hours of fasting, lipolysis (breakdown of lipids) and fat oxidation (breakdown of free fatty acids in the blood and breakdown of triglycerides in fat cells for energy) increases and blood sugar levels decrease significantly. The lipolysis increases due to lowered concentration of plasma insulin (insulin in the blood), higher concentration of growth hormone (a peptide hormone that stimulates cell reproduction, growth and cell regeneration) in the blood and increased activity of the sympathetic nervous system (stimulates to the response of fight or flight). The concentrations of plasma fatty acids (fatty acids in the blood) can increase after a fast for 14 hours (2).

The level of plasma glycerol that is based on the entire body's lipolysis, and the higher level of plasma glycerol concentration were in one study highest when individuals fasted for 12 and 24 hours. The rate of glycerol was highest after an 18 and 24 hour long fast. An increase of the fat oxidation with 50 % was showed after an 18 and 24 hour long fast. A decrease of glucose oxidation (breakdown of glucose into water and carbon dioxide) with 50 % was also showed after an 18 and 24 hour long fast.

The lower levels of plasma insulin can lead to an increase of the lipolysis due to the decrease of insulin which has the negative effect of inhibit lipolysis. In the same study described below, (2) the concentrations of plasma insulin decreased from 64.6 ± 12.9 pmol/L to 30.1 ± 7.9 pmol/L after a 12 and 72 hour long fast. 70 % decrease of plasma insulin appeared within the first 24 hours of fasting. These results are very interesting because they emerge after just an 18 and 24 hour long fast. These results show that a fast for 18 and 24 hours help the body to break down stored triglycerides and increase the fat oxidation. An increase of the lipolysis can increase fatty acid mobilization and the utilization in adipocytes (fat cells that store energy as fat) and oxidation and uptake in other tissues in the body which lead to an increase of the energy consumption which is a great factor for the treatment of obesity (2).

In another study where lean women and men fasted for 14 to 36 hours, the resting energy expenditure increased from 3.97 ± 0.9 kJ / min to 4.37 ± 0.9 kJ / min due to increased concentrations of noradrenaline. Within the fast of 14 to 36 hours there was other factors observed such as increased beta hydroxybutyrate (a ketone body involved in the metabolism of fatty acids) and plasma fatty acids as well as a decrease of the levels of triglycerides and respiratory quotient (the ratio of production of carbon dioxide to the consumption of oxygen). These factors are important for the body to utilize more fat when it is burning energy (2).

If you utilize intermittent fasting as a lifestyle you might live longer and reduce the risk of developing diseases that are common when you get older (2).

If you reduce the calorie intake and utilize intermittent fasting, the harmful effects caused by obesity such as increased insulin resistance and lowered glucose tolerance will be reduced (6). If you utilize intermittent fasting for only 12 hours each day the metabolic improvements caused by intermittent fasting will be maintained (8).

In another study, (1) 34 resistance-trained males with the age of 29.21 years ± 3.8 years and a weight of 84.6 kg (188 lbs) ± 6.2 kg (13.77 lbs) trained three times per week (Monday, Wednesday, Friday) for 8 weeks. They trained 3 sets of 6 – 8 repetitions (reps) with 85 – 90 % of 1RM (when only one rep can be done with a weight) with three minutes' rest between the sets. They were in the concentric phase (contraction that shortens a muscle) for one second and in the eccentric phase (contraction that lengthens a muscle) for two seconds. They always trained between the time 2 PM and 4 PM. Out of these 34 resistance-trained males 17 participants fasted and 17 participants ate normal food. The participants that fasted ate all their food at 1 PM, 4 PM and 8 PM and then fasted for 16 hours. The group that fasted consumed 40 % of the calories at 1 PM, 25 % of the calories at 4 PM and 35 %

of the calories at 8 PM while the group that didn't fast consumed 25 % of the calories at 8 AM, 40 % of the calories at 1 PM and 35 % of the calories at 8 PM. The participants had to consume their meals in one hour. After these 8 weeks, the group that fasted lost 16.4 % of their fat mass while the other group lost 2.8 %. Fat free mass (includes bone, internal organs, water, muscle and connective tissue, muscle mass) increased with 0.86 % in the fasted group and 0.64 % in the other group. The leg strength increased to the same level in the both groups. Testosterone (an anabolic hormone, a male sex hormone, but is also produced in women in lower levels, that is responsible for reproductive and sexual development) and IGF-1 (insulin-like growth factor 1, an anabolic hormone that is important for growth) reduced in the group that fasted but not in the other group. Blood sugar and insulin levels were reduced and HOMA-IR (homeostasis model assessment-insulin-resistance, beta-cell function and insulin resistance are quantified through this method) was improved in the group that fasted. Other metabolic changes in the group that fasted was increased adiponectin, decreased leptin, decreased T3 (is released from the thyroid gland and affects all organs and cells in the body), decreased levels of triglycerides, decreased levels of TNF-alpha (tumor necrosis factor alpha, a cell signaling protein that is responsible in the inflammation process and is also important for the acute phase reaction) and IL-1 Beta (Interleukin 1 beta, is responsible in the inflammatory response). (1).

If you utilize intermittent fasting (16 hours long fast) and exercise at the same time, you will maintain muscle mass, reduce inflammation markers, reduce body fat and reduce anabolic hormones such as IGF-1 and testosterone (1). The result of lower body fat in the recently described study above in the group that fasted is caused by the calorie deficit and the time of the day when the meals were consumed. One effect of this process is the increase of adiponectin that interacts with adenosine 5'-monophosphate-activated protein kinase (AMPK - an enzyme that is important for the homeostasis of cellular energy) and stimulates Peroxisome proliferator-activated receptor gamma co-activator 1-alpha (PGC-1 alpha, is important for the regulation of the metabolism of cellular energy) protein expression and mitochondrial biogenesis (cells increase the mass of mitochondria to increase the ATP-production to give energy). The adiponectin is also effective in the brain where it increases energy consumption which leads to weight loss (1).

In the study, testosterone and IGF-1 were reduced, but these results are not harmful for the muscles and the body composition. It is also shown in earlier studies that the concentration of testosterone is lowered in men who follows a diet and consumes less calories than the body burns in a day. The results of decreased concentrations of IGF-1 is probably caused by decreased levels of leptin and increased levels of adiponectin (1).

In this current study (1) the concentration of insulin and blood sugar reduced in the group that fasted which are good factors for the treatment of some diseases. The concentration of adiponectin did also increase and the concentration of insulin decreased which may relate to higher insulin sensitivity. Adiponectin has also a very powerful anti-inflammatory effect which leads to a reduction of inflammatory markers, and when the inflammatory markers are decreased, the relation of an improved insulin sensitivity occurs. Inflammation can be triggered of cytokines such as TNF-alpha via IKK-beta (inhibitor of nuclear factor kappa-B kinase subunit beta, is involved in the triggering of immune responses) and JNK (c-Jun-N terminal kinase, belongs to the mitogen activated protein kinase (MAPK – is important for the regulation of gene expression, cell proliferation, cell differentiation, apoptosis and cell survival) family and is responsible for cell death) / NF-kB (is important for genes involved in inflammation, immune response and cell survival) pathways which can increase the serine / threonine phosphorylation (are transmembrane proteins that bind superfamily members of growth factor beta that are transforming) of insulin receptor substrate 1 (is important for transmitting signals from receptors of IGF-1 and insulin to pathways of MAPK and intracellular pathways of protein kinase B (is important for apoptosis, glucose metabolism and cell proliferation) / PI3K (is important for cell proliferation, cell growth, cell motility, cell differentiation, intracellular trafficking and cell survival)). Furthermore, IL-6 (Interleukin 6, functions as an anti-inflammatory myokine (in response to muscular contractions, these small proteins are released by muscle cells) and a pro-inflammatory cytokine (small proteins that are important for cell signaling)) can reduce insulin sensitivity in the skeletal muscles by stimulating the toll-like-receptors-4 (TLR-4, a protein that is important for the innate immune system) gene expression through STAT3 (activator of transcription 3 and signal transducer, a transcription factor that is important for some cellular processes like apoptosis and cell proliferation) activation. This relation can activate NF-KB / IKK-beta which leads to the production of TNF-alpha (1).

The both groups in the current study had the same muscle mass after the eight weeks of training and fasting/eating normal. In mice, IGF-1 and testosterone are reduced in a calorie deficit but not in humans in the long term, instead the concentration of serum insulin-like growth factor binding protein 1 (IGFBP-1, a protein that is important for cell metabolism and cell migration and binds IGF-1 and IGF-2) is increased. Lower concentrations of IGF-1 is a good factor to reduce the risk of developing cancer but it is also a bad factor for building muscle (1). So, I believe that you have two ways to go in your life, if you want to be as healthy as possible, you should decrease the concentrations of IGF-1 for a while (losing weight) and reduce the risk of developing cancer or you can choose the other way which is building muscle and at the same time have a higher risk of developing cancer. However, the risk of cancer is decreased if you have low body fat, so maybe it is a good choice to first reduce your weight and body fat and after that build muscle until you have 12 – 14 % of body fat and then cut again and repeat this process until you have your goal weight with the goal body fat.

Intermittent fasting is also a good strategy to promote autophagy (when the body gets rid of broken cellular cells such as proteins, organelles and cell membranes) when there is no energy to fill them with. This bodily mechanism is a good strategy for optimal muscle health (1).

The study's conclusion was that intermittent fasting is a good lifestyle for athletes who want to maintain their muscle mass and lose fat at the same time (1).

In a study where the male participants had a normal bodyweight, they were forced to fast for 20 hours a day and consume food for 4 hours a day where they ate one meal during those 4 hours of the day for 8 weeks. The participants were not allowed to choose food. The food was served at the evening for 4 hours each day for 8 weeks.

The bodyweight was reduced after the 8 weeks of intermittent fasting. When the participants ate one meal a day (fast for 20 hours) the bodyweight was on average 65.9 kg (146.44 lbs) ± 3.2 kg (7.11 lbs) and when the other group of the participants ate three meals a day the bodyweight was on average 67.3 kg (149.55 lbs) ± 3.2 kg (7.11 lbs). When the participants ate one meal a day the fat mass was on average 14.2 kg (31.55 lbs) ± 1.0 kg (2.22 lbs) and after three meals a day the fat mass was on average 16.3 kg (36.22 lbs) ± 1.0 kg (2.22 lbs). After one meal per day, the fat free mass was on average 50.9 kg (113.11 lbs) ± 0.4 kg (0.88 lbs) compared with three meals per day 49.4 kg (109.77 lbs) ± 0.4 kg (0.88 lbs).

If you would consume one meal each evening after a 20 hour long fast for 8 weeks, you would increase fat free mass and reduce fat mass which are good health factors for many people.

The total cholesterol was 217 ± 5 mg/dl after one meal a day compared with 191 ± 5 mg/dl after three meals a day. The low-density lipoprotein (LDL – usually called the "bad cholesterol") was 136 ± 4 mg/dl after one meal a day compared with 113 ± 4 mg/dl after three meals a day. The high-density lipoprotein (HDL – usually called the "good cholesterol") was 62 ± 2 mg/dl after one meal a day compared with 57 ± 2 mg/dl after three meals a day. The concentrations of triglycerides were 93 ± 8 mg/dl after one meal a day compared with 102 ± 8 mg/dl after three meals a day.

The bodyweight was on average lower among the participants in the group who consumed one meal a day because they ate 65 calories less than the other group. They consumed less calories because they felt so saturated after consuming all the calories in just 4 hours a day (2).

Research shows that by utilizing intermittent fasting (fasting for 16 – 18 hours a day) you will experience increased alertness / excitement and increased mental acuity (11). This is something I love the most about intermittent fasting. When you wake up in the mornings and don't eat for 6 – 8 hours you will be more focused and driven. This is the time where I do all my work such as writing this book, searching for articles, make important phone calls, clean my apartment and of course working out. You will save so much time by not eating every 2 – 3 hours a day, instead you can fast and enjoy your life like I do.

The goal of losing weight is to minimize the loss of fat free mass and maximize body fat loss to dampen the decline in rest energy consumption and to maintain physical function which prevents weight gain (11). The goal of weight loss is also to maintain muscle mass (13). In one study made on young adult men who performed weight training and utilized intermittent fasting (fasting for 16 hours a day) for 8 weeks maintained their muscle mass, lost some fat mass and improved their muscle stamina. This study led to a conclusion that intermittent fasting combined with weight training is good for improving physical performance (11).

Chapter 8
Research of diets and macronutrients

In a study, the participants either reduced the calorie intake to 1000 or 1200 calories a day (22 participants) or reduced the fat intake to 22 or 26 grams a day (26 participants). The group that reduced the fat intake had to consume 20 % of the calories from fat on a 1000 – 1200 calorie diet which corresponds to 22 or 26 grams of fat per day. The participants were 39.2 ± 4.8 years old and 35.5 ± 5.4 years old and had a body weight of 84.5 kg (187.7 lbs) ± 8.4 kg (18.6 lbs) and 80.2 kg (178.2 lbs) ± 5.8 kg (12.8 lbs) (14).

The results of this study showed that the group that reduced the calorie intake lost 11.2 kg (24.8 lbs) ± 5.0 kg

(11.1 lbs) during the time of six months while the other group that reduced the fat intake lost 6.1 kg (13.5 lbs) ± 4.7 kg (10.4 lbs) during the time of six months. The group that reduced the calorie intake decreased the body fat percentage while the other group did not decrease the body fat percentage. The resting metabolism decreased after six months in the group that reduced the calorie intake.

These results show that a diet where the calories are reduced is more effective than a diet where the fat intake is reduced when it comes to weight loss (14).

In another study (13), the participants were ten women between the age of 23 – 39 years old and had a body fat percentage between 29 – 49 %. The study's duration was 105 days long (15 weeks). The study had two phases where the first phase was constructed to maintain the body weight. During the first phase (maintaining the body weight), the participants consumed breakfast at 8 AM – 8.30 AM and consumed 15 % of the calories during this meal, later they consumed lunch at 11.30 AM – 12 AM and consumed 35 % of the calories during this meal, further on they consumed dinner at 4.30 PM and consumed 35 % of the calories during this meal and lastly, they consumed supper at 8 PM – 8.30 PM and consumed 15 % of the calories during this meal (13).

In the second phase of the study, the first group (consumed more calories earlier in the day) consumed 35 % of the calories at breakfast and 35 % of the calories at lunch and then 15 % of the calories at dinner and 15 % of the calories at supper while the other group (consumed more calories later in the day) consumed 15 % of the calories at breakfast, 15 % of the calories at lunch, 35 % of the calories at dinner and 35 % of the calories at supper. The composition of the macronutrients was as followed: 18.1 ± 1.2 % protein, 59.7 ± 1.4 % carbohydrates and 22.3 ± 0.7 % fat. During the study the participants did some various exercises. If you want to read more about the workout regimen, you can check out the article in the references below (13).

The results showed that the group that consumed more calories earlier in the day lost more weight and fat free mass than the other group. The other group that consumed more calories later in the day lost more body fat in percentage than the other group. In the beginning of the study the group that consumed more calories later in the day had 36.3 ± 2.2 % body fat which reduced to 33.8 ± 2.3 % body fat after six weeks. The other group had 35.3 ± 2.2 % body fat in the beginning of the study which reduced to 33.5 ± 2.3 % body fat after six weeks. The group that consumed more calories later in the day lost more fat mass in phase one (13).

In phase one, the participants lost 3.79 kg (8.42 lbs) $\pm$ 0.15 kg (0.33 lbs) body weight and in phase two they lost 3.38 kg (7.51 lbs) $\pm$ 0.31 kg (0.68 lbs). In phase one, the participants lost 3.38 kg (7.51 lbs) $\pm$ 0.16 kg (0.35 lbs) fat mass and in phase two they lost 2.35 kg (5.22 lbs) $\pm$ 0.20 kg (0.44 lbs). In phase one, the participants lost 0.46 kg (1.02 lbs) $\pm$ 0.21 kg (0.46 lbs) fat free mass and in phase two they lost 1.06 kg (2.35 lbs) $\pm$ 0.20 kg (0.44 lbs) (12). The conclusion of this study was that a good weight loss is characterized by minimizing the loss of fat free mass and consuming bigger meals that contain more calories in the evening may lead to this (13).

In another study, the participants utilized a low carbohydrate diet to lose weight. Out of 891 participants only 96 participants (10.8 %) lost weight on the low carbohydrate diet (15). The participants that consumed little carbohydrates consumed more calories from fats such as monounsaturated-, saturated- and polyunsaturated fatty acids, more calories from proteins and less calories from carbohydrates than the other group that utilized a diet where carbohydrates weren't excluded. The participants that consumed less carbohydrates also exercised less than the other group. The low carbohydrate diet group also reported less hunger than the other group (15).

The low carbohydrate group lost 3.8 kg (8.4 lbs) ± 8.9 kg (19.77 lbs) of the body weight after one year, 4.5 kg (10 lbs) ± 8.0 kg (17.77 lbs) of the body weight after two years and 6.5 kg (14.4 lbs) ± 8.5 kg (18.88 lbs) of the body weight after three years while the other group that consumed more carbohydrates lost 2.3 kg (5.1 lbs) ± 5.4 kg (12 lbs) of the body weight after one year, 4.0 kg (8.8

lbs) ± 8.0 kg (17.77 lbs) of the body weight after two years and 4.7 kg (10.4 lbs) ± 9.1 kg (20.2 lbs) of the body weight after three years.

The conclusion of this study was that it isn't a big difference if you consume more carbohydrates or less carbohydrates when it comes to weight loss (15).

Like I wrote above, the goal of weight loss is to minimize the loss of fat free mass and in one study where participants consumed 22 – 29 % protein of the energy intake it resulted in less loss of fat free mass than participants that consumed 12 – 20 % protein of the energy intake (16).

The conclusion of this study made on rats was that a high protein intake is necessary for minimizing the loss of fat free mass on a diet where you eat in calorie deficit. Interestingly, the time when you consume the protein doesn't matter, this means that you can consume your protein in two meals a day or even in one meal a day (16).

In another study where protein was the main subject that was analyzed, it was showed that protein helps you feel saturated and less hungry which is associated with diet-induced thermogenesis. Protein is more saturated than fat and carbohydrates in the short- and long term. What causes the saturation effect is the activation of the thermogenesis when you consume protein. Protein is also important when it comes to body weight regulation due its effect on body composition and thermogenesis. In short term (during 24 hours) the 'fast' proteins make you feel more saturated than the 'slow' ones and protein from animals causes a higher thermogenesis than protein from vegetables. When it comes to the effect of thermogenesis and saturation in the long term, it doesn't matter what type of protein source you choose because then they have equally effects.

High protein diets are only affected on body weight loss when an individual is in calorie deficit. When more proteins are consumed in a calorie deficit, the effects are improved metabolic profile, improved body composition and lower body weight due to saturation, body composition, energy efficiency, thermogenesis and improved metabolic profile (17).

In another study conducted on both men and women, it was showed that a 500-calorie deficit (500 calories under maintenance) with either 1.6 g of protein / body weight in kg or 0.8 g of protein / body weight in kg resulted in 9.9 – 11.2 % weight loss in overweight individuals. The group that consumed 1.6 g of protein / body weight in kg lost 14.3 ± 11.8 % fat mass while the other group that consumed 0.8 g of protein / body weight in kg lost 9.3 ± 11.1 % fat mass. Interestingly, the calorie intake in both groups were the same (18).

In another study, it was showed that 15 % of protein of the total energy intake resulted in 11.4 kg (25.3 lbs) ± 3.8 kg (8.4 lbs) weight loss and 37.5 % of this weight loss was muscle mass loss. In the same study is was showed that 30 % of protein of the total energy intake resulted in 8.4 kg (18.6 lbs) ± 4.5 kg (10 lbs) weight loss and only 17.3 % of this weight loss was muscle loss.

According to this study, a protein intake of 25 – 30 % of the total energy intake is a good aiming point to protect muscle loss while in a calorie deficit (18).

It has also been proven that a higher intake of protein per body weight in kg (2.2 g / kg body weight) results in less body fat mass, decreased LDL-cholesterol and total cholesterol and decreased levels of triglycerides. This was not seen in the other group that consumed 1.1 g of protein / kg body weight.

The protein source you should consume according to this above described study is protein from animals because they have a higher amount of essential amino acids that are good for the stimulation of fat loss (18).

In a study conducted on humans it was found that participants who consumed meals after 8 PM had greater opportunities to develop increased BMI, obesity and decreased insulin sensitivity independently of when the participants went to bed or for how long they slept (19). This means that we shouldn't consume our last meal later than 8 PM.

When the diet LCHF (low carbohydrates and high fat) is utilized, almost all the carbohydrates are eliminated which results in insufficient glucose to the brain and therefore, the brain will produce ketones. Ketones make the brain work, but glucose is more efficient for the brain. LCHF will lead to decreased insulin sensitivity because the brain needs the glucose later and therefore the body saves the glucose for another occasion. Many people have barely any blood sugar when they follow the LCHF-diet, but they have high levels of insulin. When the carbohydrates are eliminated, the levels of norepinephrine and cortisol are increased, and these two hormones degrade the immune system and the muscle mass, but they also remove the carbohydrates found in the liver. Norepinephrine makes us irritated and stingy (20).

When carbohydrates are excluded from the diet, decreases the production of serotonin which is a hormone that makes us happy, calm and contributes to a good night's sleep. Too low production of serotonin can lead to an impulsive and aggressive behavior. When carbohydrates are eliminated from the diet and replaced with fat, the research shows that the risk for cardiovascular diseases increase due to increased levels of LDL. All this happens when carbohydrates are eliminated. In a study, where participants consumed either a carbohydrate-rich diet or a diet without carbohydrates, the results showed that both diets led to the same weight loss, but the participants who didn't consume carbohydrates felt more depressed than the other group (21).

When you consume your food, you should always think 'EAT SMART' which stands for Larger share of vegetables, less space for empty calories, Increase in organic growth, Proper meat and vegetable selection, Transport low (22).

The Nordic Nutrition Recommendations 2012 (NNR 2012) recommends that all individuals should increase the intake of fish and seafood, fruits and berries, nuts and seeds and vegetables and pulses. NNR 2012 also recommends that all individuals should exchange butter and butter based spreads to vegetable oils and vegetable oil based fat spreads, exchange high-fat dairy to low-fat dairy, and exchange refined cereals to wholegrain cereals. NNR 2012 also recommends all individuals to limit the intake of salt, processed meat, red meat, alcohol and beverages and foods with added sugar (23).

NNR 2012 also recommends that an unbalanced diet which does not reaches the requirements of the nutrients should NOT be complemented with supplements that contain antioxidants and vitamins for a long time because it has been showed that those supplements might increase the risk of certain adverse health effects, including mortality. Instead, the unbalanced diet should become balanced through increasing the lacking nutrients (24).

A low-energy intake is considered as an energy intake between 1552 calories and 1910 calories and these low energy intakes result in a higher risk of an insufficient intake of micronutrients (vitamins and minerals). A very low energy intake is considered as an energy intake below 1552 calories and this low energy intake is often associated with considerable risk of insufficient intake of micronutrients (24). Very low energy intakes are mainly related to a low body weight or a very low physical activity level. When an individual has a low body weight, he or she also has small muscle mass which results in a low energy expenditure. To prevent very low energy intakes and low energy intakes, NNR 2012 recommends that the physical activity level will be increased so that the individuals can consume more food and reach the requirements of the micronutrients and macronutrients and still lose body weight. For low energy intakes and very low energy intakes, NNR 2012 recommends that a multivitamin/mineral tablet is used for reaching the requirements of all the micronutrients (25).

In this chapter, I would also like to cover the importance of water. It is very important to drink enough water to feel good or else harmful consequences might occur. If you have a mild dehydration, defined as, 1 – 2 % loss of body weight due to fluid losses, the consequences might be loss of appetite, headache, vertigo and fatigue. If you have a dehydration which excess over 3 – 5 % of body weight, the consequences might be contribution to heat exhaustion and decreasing strength and endurance. If you have lost 15 – 25 % of your body weight as water, the consequences are fatal. Even if you arc consuming too much water in a short period of time, the consequences might be increased risk of hyponatremia (low levels of sodium in the blood) during pregnancy and water intoxication (26).

Chapter 9

Health benefits of physical activity

We can start with a definition of physical activity: "Physical activity includes all body movements of the skeletal muscle which results in increased energy turnover over the rest. Physical activity thus includes all body movements regardless of purpose or context". This is the definition I always use when I define physical activity, because I learned it during my education and I think it describes the whole term very good (27).

Physical activity helps to reduce the risk of chronic diseases such as cardiovascular diseases. Physical activity also helps to improve cognition, decrease the risk of depression and has a positive correlation with the body weight. Researchers say that more than 150 minutes of moderate physical activity a week may help to prevent weight gain and promote weight loss (12). Physical activity helps to improve fitness, increase muscular strength, combat cardiovascular diseases, increase lifespan and preventing diabetes type 2 (28).

In a study, where women exercised for 170 minutes a week, it was showed that they lost more weight than women who exercised for 93 and 96 minutes a week (12).

Physical activity also helps to counteract the negative consequences of obesity by reducing abdominal fat, increasing insulin sensitivity, reducing blood pressure, increasing rate of mobilization of fatty tissues, reducing subcutaneous fat, increasing metabolism and fat oxidation and increasing lipolysis activity in muscles (27).

Even more health benefits from another source is that physical activity helps to reduce the risk of certain cancers (colon cancer and breast cancer), strengthen your bones and muscles and prevent older people to fall. It is totally safe to perform moderate intensity like a quick walk, when it comes to injuries in the beginning which means that the risk of getting injured when performing moderate intensity is very low.

It is very important that you start your first time of training very slowly, because the risk of heart attacks can increase when you perform an activity very intense that you aren't used to, like running 1 mile (1.6 km) in 5 minutes. Instead, it is better to gradually increase the activity level to avoid injuries. If you have a chronic health condition such as diabetes, arthritis or heart disease, it is VERY IMPORTANT that you have a dialogue with your doctor about the training program and diet program you are about to follow. It is important that you avoid being inactive and even moderate intensity of aerobic activity like walking, running, cycling and swimming is beneficial for you (29).

On the other hand, physical inactivity with the definition "Physical inactivity includes all activities that do not lead to an energy consumption over the one that is at rest. All activities corresponding to 1.0 – 1.5 MET". Physical inactivity can be very harmful in the long term. Physical inactivity leads to the lack of muscle contractions, body fat oxidation decreases (Lipoprotein lipase decreases which catalyzes hydrolysis of triglycerides in VLDL (Very low-density lipoprotein – is a lipoprotein that is formed by apolipoproteins and cholesterol in the liver and is transporting products inside the body) and chylomicrons (lipoprotein particles that transport lipids from the diet to cardiac tissue, skeletal muscle tissue and adipose tissue) even IL-6 decreases), the amount of visceral fat increases (ectopic fat that is sensitive to inflammation), the amount of macrophages (a white blood cell that does not digest healthy body cells' proteins, instead macrophages digest foreign substances, cancer cells, cellular debris and bacteria through phagocytosis – the macrophages' digestion process), increase due to larger fat cells which lead to more proinflammatory adipokines (cytokines that promote inflammation and are excreted from immune cells such as macrophages and helper T cells – important in the adaptive immune system), systemic impact such as insulin resistance, neurodegeneration (impaired function or structure of neurons, even death of neurons), atherosclerosis (a disease where plaque is formed and the inside of an artery narrows due to the plaque) and tumor growth which may lead to cardiovascular diseases, type 2 diabetes, colon cancer, breast cancer and depression (27).

During the first six to seven weeks of strength training your strength increases due to neuronal adaptations in the nervous system. These neuronal adaptions come from improved technique when you perform the movements. When you utilize resistance training, you can expect some endocrine adjustments such as increased testosterone, growth hormone, cortisol (a steroid hormone that is secreted in response to low concentrations of blood glucose and stress, the hormone suppresses the immune system and increase blood sugar), norepinephrine, adrenaline (also known as epinephrine, is a hormone that is important in the fight-or-flight response by increasing blood sugar and blood flow to muscles), IGF-1 and insulin. IGF-1 and insulin are important for anabolic processes (when you grow and build muscles) (27).

When you utilize resistance training, you can choose to workout with free weights like barbells, dumbbells etc, or you can choose to workout with machines. Either option has advantages and disadvantages.
The benefits with strength training machines are: good muscle building, easier for beginners, steered movement, good rehabilitation and exercises training, working with thoughtful muscle, small injury risk and a great way to know the muscles (27).

The disadvantages with strength training machines are: they are rarely so well-designed that is suits all individuals, increase in strength is not transferred to sport, small/no stimulus on the stabilization muscles, slow motion, explosive strength training is difficult to implement (27).

The benefits with free weights: develops good mobility, good training for active athletes, infinite variation of each type of exercise, good muscle building, effective in both concentric and eccentric phase, develops speed and explosiveness, great stimulation on stabilization muscles, allows multi-level movements and is versatile (27).

The disadvantages with free weights: sometimes additional assistants are needed, may give lower transmission power in relation to sports momentum, main resistance in the vertical plane, in case of wrong load the damage risk increases (27).

The recommendations of physical activity according to NNR 2012 are for adults: 150 minutes of moderate intensity exercise or 75 minutes of high intensity per week. For children and adolescents: 60 minutes' moderate to very stressful physical activity per day. Everyone is recommended to reduce the sedentary (30).

When you exercise, it is important that you drink enough water because the performance begins to be affected by loss of 2 % of the body weight. If you lose 5 % of the body weight in water, your performance will be reduced with approximately 30 %.

If you don't drink enough of water, it will lead to consequences like reduced blood flow in the skin, reduced blood volume, reduced heat transfer, reduced sweat amount, increased use of muscle glycogen and increased internal temperature.

You can check your urine's color if you are in fluid balance or fluid imbalance. If you are in fluid balance the urine's color will be white and clear and if you are in fluid imbalance the urine's color will be yellow and dark yellow.

Here is a good tip on being in fluid balance before, during and after an exercise:

If you exercise in normal climate for 30 – 60 minutes then cool water is enough.

If you will exercise for a long time, like running, then you should drink 0.5 L of water 2 hours before the workout. Just before the workout you should drink 0.5 L of water. During the workout, you should drink 120 – 180 ml of water every 15 – 20 minute. After the workout, you should drink 150 % or more of the weight loss but not all at once of course (28).

If you exercise regularly then you could think about these factors: what are my meals before, during and after training / competition? Am I in energy balance (maintaining the body weight)? Do I have strategies about fluid? Do I have a good meal timing? Do I need additions? Is there something I should not eat / drink in connection with exercise? Do I have good general knowledge of nutrition? (28).

Chapter 10

Sleep recommendations

Sleep is very important for your health. If you don't sleep the hours you need per day then your health will be affected negatively. The National Sleep Foundation writes that if you, for example, sleep for 4 – 5 hours a day for a long time then your health will be affected negatively (31).

Here are the recommendations of how much sleep you need according to National Sleep Foundation:

If you are 14 – 17 years old your recommended sleep per day is 8 – 10 hours.
If you are 18 – 25 years old your recommended sleep per day is 7 – 9 hours.
If you are 26 – 64 years old your recommended sleep per day is 7 – 9 hours.
If you are older than 65 years old your recommended sleep per day is 7 – 8 hours (31).

Chapter 11

Physiology

In this chapter, I will write about how the body, mostly the gastrointestinal tract (GI), works and is structured. This will give you a better understanding of how you work as a human being. When I have written about the physiology I will go right over to the nutrition part where I will write about vitamins, minerals, carbohydrates, proteins and fats so you get a clearer understanding of how these nutrients affect your body. So, let's start with the physiology.

The GI and the digestion process

The GI is almost the same thing as the digestion process, where both are around 7 – 10 m from the lips to rectum. In the GI, we can find pharynx (pharynx), esophagus, liver (hepar), stomach (ventriculus – fundus, corpus, antrum, (parts in the stomach)), gallbladder (vesical fellea), pancreas, the small intestine (duodenum, jejunum and ileum, parts in the small intestine), colon (colon, caecum, colon ascendens, colon transversum, colon descendens and colon sigmoideum, parts in the colon), rectum and appendix (32). The words in the brackets are the Latin name of the organs and parts that are included in that specific organ, for example, colon, where the names in the brackets are parts of the colon.

There are four different processes in the GI; digestion (where different nutrients are digested by the organs), secretion (HCl (Hydrochloric acid), bile, bicarbonate, enzymes and saliva), absorption (where different nutrients are absorbed by the organs) and peristaltic, motility (transport and mixes the food forward in the digestion process) (32).

The digestion process is controlled autonomously. The first checkpoint in the digestion process is **salivation**. The saliva contains of mucus (mucin) that binds water which make the saliva slimy. The saliva is built up by 99 % of water, mucin, Ca^{2+} (calcium ions), PO_4^{3-} (phosphate), bicarbonate, saliva amylase (ptyalin - which breaks down starch), immunoglobulins, lysozyme, tongue lipase (not from spotting glands). The enzyme alpha-amylase can only break down carbohydrates and not fat and protein. The saliva is antibacterial (32). You get more saliva when you see, taste, think, smell food and have food in the mouth. The autonomic nervous system controls the salivary secretion; the parasympathetic nervous system (has the opposite effect of the sympathetic nervous system and when the fight-and-flight response is gone, the parasympathetic nervous system is activated) makes the saliva aqueous and the sympathetic nervous system makes the saliva viscous (32). The GI is mostly controlled by nerve vagus while the salivation is stimulated by XII and IX cranial nerves. There are also three pairs of spotting glands which are glandular mandibularis (longer in the mouth), glandula sublingualis (under the tongue) and glandula parotis (up in the palate and here is the most saliva produced – maximum production is 4 ml / min). The salivary glands produce around 1500 ml saliva per day. When you chew, it costs 1 – 2 % of the energy intake (33).

The second checkpoint in the digestion process is **the esophagus and upper mouthpiece**. When you swallow, you involve 14 muscle groups. When you swallow, the trachea closes. The entire esophagus is 20 – 25 cm long. The food we eat transports through the esophagus via peristaltic waves which takes about 10 seconds. This means that we can stand on the head and drink and eat because the food will be squeezed down. When you have swallowed the food, it won't go back up again because the lower sphincter is in conjunction with the cardia (33).

The third checkpoint in the digestion process is **the stomach (ventriculus)**. The stomach's volume is around 50 – 1500 ml. In the stomach, there is 0.1 M HCl, a H^+ / K^+ - ATPase-parietal (the hydrochloric acid is transported via parietal cells). In the stomach, there is also a hydrogen ion / potassium ion-antiport pump which is blocked with drugs when the acid is overproduced (31). Fundus is the top part of the stomach, body is the middle part (secretes HCl, pepsinogen and mucus), and antrum is the bottom part (secretes pepsinogen, mucus and gastrin) (32)

Via the pylorus sphincter, the stomach make 3 – 4 emptyings per minute. The transport through the stomach takes around 40 minutes for fluid and around 2 hours for food that is not fluid. The stomach also contains 8 pepsins from chief cells which are Pepsin A, B, C (gastricsin) and D (chymosin). There is also a factor called intrinsic factor that binds vitamin B12 in the stomach by producing REM proteins that take the vitamin B12 into the duodenum and release it there so intrinsic factor can binds vitamin B12 instead.

Some personal trainers without enough education says that eating raw protein gives you a better absorption in the body. This is a very bad argument and it is super false, because all protein that you consume will be destroyed in the stomach by the hydrochloric acid.
In the stomach, there is a protection of about 0.3 mm which make the absorption of the food slower but the tissue will be protected (33).

The exocrine glands in the stomach mix gastric juice with food (kymus). The gastric juice consists of HCl and intrinsic factor, pepsinogen (chief cells), mucin (mucin producing cells and bicarbonate), somatostatin (D cells) and histamine (ECL-cells).
Pepsin is activated from pepsinogen when HCl is present. Pepsin is a protease that breaks down proteins. The secretion of HCl is stimulated by histamine and gastrin and is inhibited by somatostatin (32).

The food in the stomach is transported forward by peristaltic. The pacemaker cells provide three spontaneous repolarizations / depolarizations every minute, this is the electrical rhythm in the stomach. If the stomach doesn't receive stimuli from hormones or nerves the food won't transport forward. When we consume more food in a sitting (intermittent fasting) the stomach receives stronger contractions (more action potentials) which can transport the food further. In the fundus part of the stomach, the peristaltic waves begin. When the food reaches the antrum part of the stomach, small amounts of kymus are squeezed through the pylorus sphincter into the duodenum. When both the pylorus sphincter and antrum part are contracted, the food is being mixed. The rate of the emptying of the stomach's content to the duodenum depends on what the food contains. The kymus can be absorbed and broken down with the help of nerve signals in the enteric nervous system and hormone secretion from the small intestine (32).

The fourth checkpoint in the digestion process is **the duodenum**. The duodenum is 20 cm long with a pH of 7 – 8. The pH in the stomach was 1. In the duodenum, there are a lot of releases of exocrine pancreas: lipase + co-lipase (binds to lipase that cleaves the fat), acinar (zymogenes), RNases, alpha-amylases, DNases, chymotrypsin, trypsin (activated via enterokinase) and carboxypeptidase.

The release from the ductus is bicarbonate and the releases from the vesica felleae are gall salts that break down fatty acids and fat substances.

In the duodenum, there is a 0.2 mm mucus layer as protection (33).

The fifth checkpoint in the digestion process is **the upper small intestine (jejunum)**. The jejunum is approximately 1 m long with a strong surface enlargement that is built up by folds, villi (0.5 – 1 mm; 10 – 40 mm^2), microvilli (brush border). The exocrine cells release amylase and aminopeptidases. The enzymatic activity in the brush borders are various sugar-slimming enzymes.

In the jejunum, there is a 0.15 mm mucus layer as protection (33).

The sixth checkpoint in the digestion process is **the lower small intestine (ileum)**. The surface is smaller than the jejunum. The food transports through the entire small intestine in about 3 – 5 hours. A large part of the bile salts reuptake happens in the ileum. In the lower ileum, the absorption of vitamin B12 occurs. The receptors of the intrinsic factor are also found in ileum.

In the ileum, there is a 0.5 mm mucus layer as protection (33).

The entire small intestine is strongly wrapped with villi (bowel duct) and with epithelial cells with microvilli on its surface. It is the epithelial cells that absorb nutrients with an absorption area of around 200 m^2 in an adult person.

The small intestine secretes around 1500 ml of intestinal juice every day that contain Na^+ (sodium ions), HCO3 (bicarbonate), Cl (chlorine), water and mucus (protects the epithelial cells against the enzymes in the digestion process). The small intestine breaks down proteins, carbohydrates and fats with the help of enzymes in bile and microvilli and pancreatic enzymes.

When the small intestine is moving, it is called motility and it happens in different segments so called segmentation. This segmentation happens with pacemaker rhythm. In ileum, there is nine contractions per minute and in duodenum, there is 12 contractions per minute. When the small intestine is moving, the (kymus) mixes and moves forward against the colon (32).

The seventh checkpoint in the digestion process is **the colon**. The (kymus) comes in to the colon through a sphincter. In the colon, you have a large part of your bacterial flora. In the colon, short-chain fatty acids (SCFA) such as butyric acid, propanoic acid and butanoic acid are produced. These SCFA:s are the enterocytes favorite food (33). The SCFA:s are produced when fibers don't break down by the bacteria (32). In the colon, the water is mostly absorbed. I have forgotten to mention the mask-shaped attachment and the appendix, but these have no importance for the digestion process.

In the colon, there is a 0.8 mm mucus layer as protection. The mucus layer makes the food absorption slower but it protects the colon from wound injuries because the water content has decreased and this makes the food harder and can damage the intestine (33).

Via the ileocecal sphincter, the kymus reaches the cecum (the beginning to the colon). This sphincter relaxes after every meal and closes of the extent of the colon to prevent the kymus to go backwards. Around 1500 ml of kymus per day is reduced to around 200 – 250 g feces every day. For around 18 – 24 hours, the kymus is transported in the colon. In the colon, vitamin K is produced by the bacteria. The bacteria in the colon can't go into the body because there is a lymphatic tissue in the intestinal wall (32).

Every 30 minutes, the colon is moving, called segmentation which is stimulated by the parasympathetic nervous system and inhibits by the sympathetic nervous system. Two to four times per day, there is so called mass movements in the colon that occurs after each meal. The contractions (segmentation) happens in the first part of the colon where the colon squeezes the kymus against the anus (32).

The last checkpoint in the digestion process is **the rectum**. 2 – 3 times per day, the rectum fills up by strong peristaltic waves. Two muscle layers control the anus, one interior that is controlled autonomous and one outer cross-sectional that is controlled by the human being's will. All types of broken down food are transported via the hepatic portal system to the liver except for the vascular system (33).

The rectum is usually empty, but when the walls of the rectum are stretched which happens when the kymus gets there, the defects of reflexes start which cause the kymus in the colon sigmoideum (the last part of the colon) and the entire rectum to contract at the same time. When the inner anal sphincter relaxes, we must go to the toilet and do our needs. If you do not make your needs at the time when kymus is in the rectum, it will transport back to the colon sigmoideum with the help of antiperistaltic movements. The kymus can only leave the anus when the external anal sphincter relaxes. It is not good to not do your needs when the kymus is in the rectum, because when the kymus goes back to the colon sigmoideum, it will get harder and it will hurt in the anus when you must do your needs the next time. This can be very painful in the long term because your stomach can be affected negatively. So, when you need to go to the toilet, you should go to the toilet to avoid these stomach problems (32).

Another organ in the GI is the liver or so called hepar in Latin. The liver secretes and produces bicarbonate and bile to the small intestine, the liver takes care of nutrients after they have been absorbed. The liver converts vitamin D into Calcitriol, and produces IGF-1, angiotensinogen, cholesterol, plasma proteins and coagulation factors like fibrinogen and prothrombin. The liver also disables and converts a lot of substances such as drugs, hormones and toxins.

The liver weights around 1.5 kg (3.33 lbs) and is provided with blood from the portal vein from the intestine and from the artery hepatica. All the absorbed nutrients in the blood from the GI passes the liver through vena cava inferior before it reaches the rest of the body (32).

In the body, we produce and supply water to make the GI function well. We supply approximately 2 L of water to the GI per day. We produce approximately 1.5 L of saliva per day, 2.5 L of gastric juice, 1.5 L of pancreas, 0.5 L of bug. This equals 8 L. 6.5 L of this amount is taken up in the small intestine and 1.3 L is taken up in the large intestine. Through the drainage, we lose around 0.2 L of liquid (33).

The GI is affected by hormones in the body. For example, gastrin, a hormone released from antrum and duodenum, that stimulates antrum contraction, acid secretion, small intestine motility. It inhibits the sphincter between the colon and the ileum. Gastrin is released by peptides and amino acids in the stomach and it is inhibited by somatostatin and secretin.
Somatostatin, another hormone that is released from the endocrine pancreas that inhibits small intestine and stomach hyperplasia and gall bladder contraction.
GIP (gastric inhibitory peptide), another hormone that stimulates insulin release and inhibits motility in the stomach.

Cholecystokinin (CCK) is a peptide that is released from mucosal cells in the duodenum. CCK is released by fatty acids and amino acids in the duodenum. CCK stimulates enzyme secretion pancreas, bicarbonate secretion, gall bladder contraction and relaxes Sphincter Oddi.

Secretin is also a peptide that is released from mucosal cells in the duodenum. Secretin is released by acid in the duodenum. Secretin collaborates with CCK and it also stimulates bicarbonate secretion from the liver and the pancreas (33).

The human body + energy

If a person is 25 years old and weights 70 kg (155.55 lbs), he or she consists of 42 kg (93 lbs) water of which 14 kg (31.1 lbs) extracellular fluid (the fluid outside the cells) and 28 kg (62.2 lbs) intracellular fluid (the fluid inside the cells).

The human body's energy storage is built up by 2 – 3 kg (4.44 – 6.66 lbs) of protein which is around 10.000 calories, 12 kg (26.66 lbs) of fat which is around 90.000 calories and less than 1 kg (2.22 lbs) of carbohydrates which is around 4.500 calories. This energy storage means that the human body can live without food for a maximum of two months (6).

The human body consists of bone that is built up by crystalline calcium phosphate (hydroxyapatite), 1 kg (2.22 lbs) of calcium and ½ kg (1.11 lbs) of phosphorus. In the skeleton, there is half of the body's collagen (6).

The human body also consists of muscles where 40 % of the body weight is skeletal muscle, 10 % of the body weight is smooth muscle and very little of the body weight is cardiac muscle. The muscle cells contain a lot of water, approximately 75 % of water (6).

The human body also consists of 5 liters of blood where of 45 % is cell mass (hematocrit) and 55 % is plasma. The oxygen carrying capacity in the human body is 200 ml oxygen / liter excluding erythrocytes which has 3 ml oxygen / liter (6).

The human body consists of, like I mentioned before, 12 kg (26.66 lbs) of fat which is around 17 % of the body weight for a person that weights 70 kg (155.55 Ibs). There is 90 % of subcutaneous fat + part of the abdominal cavity. 2 kg (4.44 lbs) are essential and 10 kg (22.2 lbs) are stored (90.000 calories which is around 4 weeks of storage) (6).

In the human body, there is brown fatty tissue that is mitochondrial dietary fat cells. When the fat from the brown fatty tissue is needed, it will be activated very quickly to be used. The brown fatty tissue helps to generate heat through uncouplers which is a chemical efficiency (6).

If we leave the content of the human body and go over to the body composition (body weight, BMI (Body Mass Index), fat mass, water percentage, muscle mass and bone mass). It is sometimes good to measure the body composition to get a better understanding if you are overweight or underweight. When the body composition is analyzed, it will provide clues about hydrogenation changes like edema, diarrhea, marasmus, kwashiorkor, kidney or cardiac damage (6).

To measure the body composition, you can choose some alternatives, but I will only describe two of them, which I think is the most important and the best to choose. The first alternative is weighting + measuring which will give you a number that is your BMI. To be healthy according to the BMI, you will have a BMI between 20 and 25. To calculate the BMI you simply take your body weight in kg (lbs x 0.45 = kg) and divide this with your length in meters' times two. So, for example, I am 173 cm tall, which means I will divide my weight with 1.73 x 1.73 = 2.9929. This gives me the body weight in kg divided with 2.9929 which gives the number of my BMI.

The formula for the BMI is (body weight in kg / length in meters x length in meters).

There is one weakness with this method and it is that you will have a high BMI (over 25) if you are very muscular which means that you are obese, but in fact, you are not (6).

The second alternative is a DEXA (Dual-Energy X-ray Absorptionmetry) scan which measures three compartments at once (soft tissue, bone and fat). This is the most precious method in the world that measures your body composition (6).

I haven't used the DEXA scan, instead, I use a person scale that measures the body weight, BMI, body fat percentage, water percentage in the body, muscle mass percentage and bone mass in kg. Here, you don't have to calculate your BMI, because the scale does it on its own, you just must give it your length and your body weight. You can buy these types of scales at the electronic store (6).

Contribution to energy consumption

When we are at rest, our bodies burn calories. This is because the cells in our bodies are working and makes us burn calories. This is called basal metabolism (how many calories the body expends when it is in rest). The basal metabolism is also affected by sex and age. When we break down the food we have eaten, it affects the energy consumption with around 10 %. Around 30 % of the total energy consumption comes from physical activity (6).

The basal metabolism is controlled by age (it is at its peak around 20 – 25 years old and after that age, the basal metabolism decreases), body surface (a taller and slimmer person has a higher basal metabolism than a shorter and thicker person), growth (when you get more muscles from working out or you get pregnant, you become bigger and this affects the basal metabolism with around 5 calories / gram newly formed tissue), constitution (the more muscles you have the more calories you will burn because muscle cells burn more calories than fat cells), fever (if your body temperature increases with one degree Celsius, the basal metabolism increases with 10 %), climate (if it is cold outside the basal metabolism raises because the body need to maintain the body temperature, moderate heat decreases and extremely heat raises), fasting lowers the basal metabolism (6).

The basal metabolism is also affected by different forms of thermogenesis (the mechanism of production of heat in organisms) like isometric thermogenesis (when the muscle tension is increased but no work is done), dynamic thermogenesis (when you stretch your muscles or when you climb down a ladder), psychological thermogenesis (like expectations, anxiety, stress which stimulates secretion of adrenaline), diet-induced thermogenesis (if you eat spicy food or a lot of carbohydrates you will get warm and burn more calories) and medicine-induced thermogenesis (coffee raises the metabolism with 5 – 10 % over two hours, tea also raises the metabolism) (6).

Chapter 12
Nutrition (macronutrients and micronutrients)

I will begin to describe some of the most important micronutrients that we need to consume every day.

Micronutrients are the name for vitamins and minerals and means micro = small amount, and nutrients = categories of food that the human can consume. I will begin to describe some minerals that are important for the body.

The recommendations (the recommended intake) of all the macronutrients and micronutrients are based on different types of scientific evidence and these recommendations are made to assure optimal development and function in the body and contribute to a decreased risk of major chronic diseases (34).

Sodium as salt

Sodium is mainly found in processed foods like cheese, bread, meat, spreads and fish products. Salt and sodium chloride (NaCl) are nutritionally equivalent (35).
The sodium ion is important for the regulation of the osmotic pressure in the extracellular fluid volume, the acid-base balance, nerve function, blood volume, the transport of certain amino acids and glucose and is also

important for some metabolic processes in the cell. In the body, there is around 100 grams of sodium in an adult and the half of this amount is found in the extracellular fluid volume. Around 10 grams of the body pool of sodium is found in cells. The rest of the sodium is found in the skeleton. Around 90 % of the sodium from the diet is absorbed in the body and around 100 – 200 mmol of sodium is excreted effectively through the kidneys and the skin daily. 99.5 % of the sodium can be retained in the body through the tubule cells in the kidneys. A lot of sodium can also be excreted through the kidneys. For this to happen, a sufficient supply of water is needed because the concentration of the urine is limited. It also requires healthy kidneys (36).

Deficiency of sodium can occur when a person is sweating heavy and is not consuming sodium. Deficiency of sodium can also occur in connection with prolonged diarrhea and vomiting without consumption of sodium. The symptoms of deficiency of sodium is loss of appetite, muscle seizures and disturbances of the circulation and if there is a severe deficiency, the consequences might be death and coma. The sodium balance can be maintained by 0.6 grams of salt per day but the lowest recommended intake for salt is 1.5 grams per day, but this recommendation will vary depending on the climate and physical activity (36,37).

A lower intake of sodium as salt is very beneficial for the human body. A reduced intake of sodium as salt results in decreased blood pressure and decreased risk of cardiovascular mortality and morbidity (38).

Recommendations of sodium and salt

The recommended intake for sodium for the person over 10 year of age is 2.4 grams per day and the recommended intake for salt for the person over 10 year of age is 6 grams per day (35). The lowest recommended intake for salt is 1.5 grams per day, but this recommendation will vary depending on the climate and physical activity (37).

Calcium

Calcium is most important for our bones and teeth, but also neuronal contractions and muscle contractions (1 % of the calcium is needed for the contractions) (39). In the body, we find 99 % of the calcium in our bones (in the form of hydroxyapatite) and teeth and the rest is found in extracellular fluid, blood and in all body's cells. The free calcium is important for signal transduction between cells and within cells, glandular secretion, neuromuscular transmission and in enzymatic reactions. Calcium is regulated by two hormones which are 1,25-dihydroxyvitamin D_3 ($1,25(OH)_2D$) and parathyroid hormone (40). When we consume the calcium, it is in the form of hydroxyapatite. Around 14 % of our body weight is bone mass where the most weight is in the legs and arms (39).

Calcium in the digestive juices are mixed with dietary calcium in the intestine, and this mixture of calcium is absorbed in the upper part of the ileum with the help of an active energy requiring process or passive diffusion. If you have vitamin D deficiency, the absorption of calcium will be decreased. The net absorption of calcium is around 34 % during puberty when the energy intake is 925 milligrams per day (41,42).

If we don't consume enough calcium (hypocalcaemia) it can lead to tetany which is a form of involuntary muscle contractions that hurt. If we on the other hand consume too much calcium (hypercalcemia) it can cause you to feel thirsty, confused, weak and less hungry.

When you are between 18 and 25 years old, it is very important to consume enough calcium (around 130 – 160 mg per day of calcium) to reduce the risk of osteoporosis (weakness of the bones can lead to the development of a broken bone) (39).

When we are younger we have more osteoblasts in our body and when we get older we have more osteoclasts in our body. Osteoblasts build up the bone and osteoclasts break down the bone. Therefore, many older people have a higher risk of developing osteoporosis (39).

When we consume calcium, it is absorbed to 15 – 80 %
in the duodenum and ileum. After the absorption in the
duodenum and ileum, the absorbed calcium goes out in
the blood and transports to the bones, teeth and a lot goes
to the kidneys (39). We lose calcium through the skin,
feces and urine and if you consume around 1,000
milligrams of calcium per day, then around 70 % - 80 %
will be lost (42).

The absorption of calcium increases through free fatty
acids and lactose but also of an enough intake of vitamin
D.
The absorption of calcium decreases through stress, the
older you get, medicines, phytic acid and oxalic acid in
plant foods and phosphates.
A high intake of protein and sodium leads to a negative
effect on the secretion of calcium (39).

The risk group of calcium deficiency is the people who
are lactose intolerant.
Osteoporosis is something that is associated with calcium
deficiency, and this is something you know after you

have read the above written sentences, but osteoporosis can also be caused by a high intake of alcohol, the people who consumed very little calories in their young ages, people who are smoking, diabetes, low physical activity and low BMI.

A very interesting thing is that if you are born in Africa, you have a lower risk of developing osteoporosis (39).

You can find calcium in all milk products, fishes with bones (small fishes), soybean products (tofu), yoghurt, cheese, products with low fat percentage that you can have in the fridge (39).

Recommendations of calcium

The recommended intake for both men and women is 800 milligrams per day. The lowest recommended intake for both men and women is 400 milligrams per day. The highest recommended intake for both men and women is 2,500 milligrams per day (40).

Potassium

98 % of the potassium is found intracellular and is the most important positive ion (cation) intracellular. 2 % of the potassium is found extracellular (outside the cells) and functions as a regulator for the membrane potential of the cells, and therefore, it is important for blood pressure regulation, muscle and nerve function and the acid-base balance.

You can find potassium in fruits and berries, milk and dairy products, potatoes and vegetables.

90 % of the potassium from dietary intake is absorbed from the gut and the potassium is lost through the urine and sweat. Through prolonged vomiting and diarrhea and the use of diuretics and laxatives, deficiency of potassium can occur. It is uncommon to get deficiency of potassium because there is potassium in many food products. Hereditary defects in renal salt transporters like Gitelman's syndrome and Bartter's syndrome, hyperaldosteronism (a too high production of aldosterone in the adrenal glands), excessive consumption of licorice increases potassium excretion and sodium retention

which all can result in hypokalemia (the levels of potassium ions are too low in the blood serum). The symptoms of potassium deficiency are mental disturbances like confusion and depression, disturbed function of the cell membrane which can result in muscle weakness and disturbances in the function of the heart which can result in heart seizure and arrhythmia. The blood pressure can be increased in both people with normal blood pressure (normotensive) and people with high blood pressure (hypertensive) if the intake of potassium is too low because a too low intake of potassium can induce sodium retention (43,44).

Potassium can decrease the blood pressure and might reduce the risk of cardiovascular endpoints and stroke (45).

Potassium chloride tablets have been associated with acute poisoning in humans! Symptoms that have been reported are cyanosis (a too low oxygen saturation in the tissues near the skin's surface which gives the skin a purple or blue color), heart failure, cardiac arrest, nausea, diarrhea, abdominal pain, vomiting, ulceration of the stomach, ileum, duodenum and esophagus (46).

Potassium from the food have not been associated with negative effects in humans, but a too high intake of potassium for a long period of time might result in hyperkalemia (the levels of potassium ions are too high in the blood serum) with symptoms like impaired function of the kidneys and affected functions of the heart (46).

Recommendations of potassium

The recommended intake for men is 3.5 grams per day and for women 3.1 grams per day of potassium. The lowest recommended intake for potassium is 1.6 grams per day for both men and women (43).

Phosphorus

In the body, there is between 800 grams to 1200 grams of phosphorus and of these 800 – 1200 grams, 85 % is in the skeleton and the other 15 % is distributed in all tissues. About 1 % of the total body mass is comprised by phosphate (47). Phosphorus is responsible for the energy metabolism, nucleic acids, phospholipids, the production of the collagen (39) cell structure, bone mineralization, regulation of subcellular processes, cellular metabolism and maintenance of acid-base homeostasis (47).

The absorption of phosphorus can be increased by a high intake of vitamin D (39).

The body phosphorus content is regulated by two compounds called fibroblast growth factor 23 and Klotho together with parathyroid hormone, and these are released when phosphorus is consumed in the body. By the epithelium of the jejunum and duodenum in the small intestine, dietary phosphate is absorbed through passive diffusion. Calcitriol is regulated by serum phosphate, when phosphate decreases, the production of calcitriol increases. The absorption of phosphate is regulated by the sodium dependent phosphate transporters' function, especially NaPiIIb whose activity is regulated by calcitriol.

The absorption is between 55 % and 70 % in adults when the diet is mixed.

In the kidney, NaPiIIa is the main sodium dependent phosphate transporter which is regulated by fibroblast growth factor 23, Klotho, parathyroid hormone and dietary phosphate (48,49).

If you eat too little of phosphorus you can get problems with the muscles, anorexia, dizziness and decalcification of the skeleton (39), rickets (soft or weak bones in children), impaired bone mineralization, the nervous system, the function of the kidney and osteomalacia (soft bones). It is though very uncommon to get deficiency symptoms of phosphorus (49). On the other hand, if you eat too much of phosphorus you can get diarrhea, convulsions, kidney and bone damage, vascular calcification, premature ageing and soft tissue calcification (39).

The risk group of phosphor deficiency is premature children and people who are anorexians.
You can find phosphorus in legumes, milk, meat and grain products (48).

Recommendations of phosphorus

The recommended intake of phosphorus for both men and women is 600 milligrams per day. The lowest recommended intake is 300 milligrams per day for both men and women. The highest recommended intake is 3,000 milligrams per day for both men and women (47).

Magnesium

Around 20 – 60 % of the magnesium from the diet is absorbed in the body. Magnesium is important for gene regulation, energy-dependent membrane transport, transmission of neuromuscular impulses and sustained electrical potential in nerves and cell membranes. In the body, the adult human has around 20 – 28 grams of magnesium where 40 – 45 % is intracellular in soft tissues and muscles, 1 % is extracellular and the rest is in the skeleton (50,51).

Magnesium is important for neurons and muscle cells, cofactor in the energy metabolism and replication of DNA and RNA (39).

If you consume too little magnesium you can get hypercalcemia (the levels of calcium ions are too high in the blood serum), hypokalemia, electrocardiographic abnormalities, neuromuscular hyper excitability and cardiac arrhythmias. After 78 days of an intake of 101 milligrams per day of magnesium adverse heart rhythm changes have been observed (51). If you instead consume too much magnesium (0.5 – 5 grams/day) you can get diarrhea (39).

The risk group of magnesium deficiency is people who have diabetes, drink too much alcohol and have renal diseases. Unless you don't fall into any of these categories, you can feel calm, because it is very hard to get magnesium deficiency. This means that buying a magnesium supplement is a waste of money (39).

You can find high concentrations of magnesium in nuts, dark chocolate and coffee. You can also find magnesium in green leafy vegetables, whole grain cereals and legumes (50).

Recommendations of magnesium

The recommended intake for men is 350 milligrams per day and for women 280 milligrams per day (50).

Iron

The world's highest deficiency of any mineral is iron. Iron takes care of the oxygen transport by creating the oxygen-binding part of hemoglobin (hemoglobin from lungs to blood and myoglobin for muscle fibers). Iron is also important for ATP formation, cytochrome enzyme, peroxidase, catalase and the electron transport chain because iron can be in the form of 2^+ (ferrous iron) or 3^+ (ferric iron). Heme iron is in the form of 2^+ while non-heme iron is in the form of 3^+. The heme iron is always bounded to the structure of hemoglobin while non-heme iron is bounded to other proteins during the transport in the electron transport chain (52). In the body, iron can be stored as hemosiderin and ferritin which are storage proteins in the spleen, liver and bone marrow. You can also find very small amounts of ferritin in plasma in the form of an iron-free form (53).

Around 2-3-5 % of the iron is absorbed in the small intestine and is transported with transferrin to different places in the body like the bone marrow where the erythropoiesis (the production of red blood cells) takes place, the liver and the cell tissue. The iron is destroyed in the spleen and this is how the iron goes around in the body.

The iron intake should increase with around 20 % when girls have their periods, during pregnancy and growth. The human body can't secrete iron and this means that it is very easy to overdo iron (52). The iron is maintained in the body through regulators such as small peptide hepcidin (encoded by the HAMP-17 gene) that is expressed in the liver (53). The only way iron can leave the body though is from bleedings and through skin cells that are being destroyed, therefore it is very easy to overdo iron and that is very unhealthy (52).

Iron in foods in the form of heme iron is easier absorbed than iron in the form of non-heme iron and the iron is absorbed better if it comes from animal products (contain heme iron) than plant products (contain non-heme iron) (52). If a person has iron deficiency, the absorption is better than if a person doesn't have iron deficiency (53). Around 25 % of heme iron from food is absorbed in the body.

The uptake of iron is inhibited when we consume calcium from milk (one glass of milk which contains about 165 mg of calcium reduces the absorption of iron with 50 %), cacao, phosphates, phytates, iron-binding polyphenols like tannins, large amounts of manganese, bran and coffee and tea (contain iron-binding polyphenols). Intakes above 300 milligrams of calcium won't increase further reduction of the absorption of iron. Calcium through supplementation also reduces the absorption of iron (54).

The uptake of iron is stimulated when we consume vitamin C with the largest effect of intakes up to 100 milligrams per day of ascorbic acid (you can find vitamin

C in vegetable salad, fresh vegetables, fresh berries and fruits and fruit juice), acetic acid added to dough (low pH), meat, poultry and fish (which all three products include a factor called MFP-factor) because iron in the form of 3^+ is converted into the iron of 2^+ which makes it easier for the human body to consume it (52).

We need some extra iron when we are growing, during pregnancy and during lactation (52).

A too high intake of iron is deadly for children because it can lead to hepatic necrosis (loss of the liver's functions). It gets deadly when you consume $180 - 300$ mg per kg body weight.

You can get a disease from iron that is deadly and is called hemochromatosis and means that the absorption of the iron is too high in the body which can lead to poisoning. People who have this disease must get rid of free iron ions in the blood that are toxic to the body (52).

An acute overdose of preparations of pharmaceutical iron results in mucosal erosion in the intestine and stomach, which can lead to a very high absorption of iron due to damage to the intestinal mucosa, and the symptoms from this can be heart failure, capillary leakage and vascular dilatation. Organs like the pancreas, liver, red blood cells, central nervous system and kidney can also be damaged by the iron. Other symptoms are heartburn, vomiting, nausea and epigastric discomfort like occasional diarrhea and constipation (55).

If you consume too little iron, you can get iron deficiency anemia and the symptoms are exhaustion, tiredness, paleness, headache, reduced work capacity, impaired immune response and impaired cognitive functions in children.
You can find iron in cereals, black pudding, meat and whole grains (52).

Recommendations of iron
The recommended intake of iron for men is 9 milligrams per day. The recommended intake of iron for women in the age between 19 – 50 years is 15 milligrams per day and the recommended intake for women in the age

between 51 – 75+ is 9 milligrams per day. The lowest recommended intake is 7 milligrams per day for men and for women in the age between 51 – 75+ 5 milligrams per day. The highest recommended intake for both men and women is 60 milligrams per day.

Women in the age between 19 – 50 years need more iron because they lose iron through menstrual bleeding and the transfer of iron to the fetus when they are pregnant (56).

Zinc

More than 300 enzymes need zinc and therefore zinc is a coenzyme to many enzymes. Zinc is responsible for the prostate, vision, normal production of DNA, function of the immune system, cell division, protection of lipids and proteins from oxidative damage, cognitive function, maintenance of normal bone density, reproduction, fertility, acid-base metabolism, metabolism of vitamin A and fatty acids, protein metabolism, cell membrane, pancreas (the production and action of insulin) and nucleic acid production (57). Zinc seems also to stimulate insulin receptor tyrosine kinase activity and insulin action (58,59).

In the upper part of the small intestine, the absorption of zinc mainly occurs. Zinc is transported with transferrin and mainly albumin in the blood circulation. Most of the zinc (2 – 4 grams) is in the cells. Around 66 % of the zinc is found in muscle tissue and around 33 % is found in bone tissue. Zinc in plasma is estimated to be around 0.1 % of the total zinc content. In prostate liquid and in parts of the eye, there is high concentrations of zinc. Zinc is lost through the skin, kidneys and GI. Zinc is maintained in the body through strong homeostatic mechanisms. Zinc deficiency is thought to be high in many countries in Africa and Asia and countries that are thought to have low risk of developing zinc deficiency are countries in North America and Europe. The symptoms of severe zinc deficiency are delayed sexual maturation, growth retardation, hair loss, skin lesions adjacent to the body orifices and behavioral disturbances. These symptoms have almost only been observed in people with acrodermatitis enteropathica which is a problem in the transport of zinc, and in adolescents that do not consume enough of zinc. Zinc is used in countries where there is zinc deficiency as a pharmacological agent against chronic diarrhea (58).

The human body absorbs around 15 – 40 % of the zinc. People who are fasting, has anorexia, are in periods of tissue growth, are lactating or are pregnant need more zinc and people who has fever or an infection need less zinc (52)

The absorption of zinc is stimulated by animal protein (20 – 40 % of the zinc is absorbed) and inhibited of phytic acid (found in cereals and leguminous plants) (10 – 15 % of the zinc is absorbed) and iron. Zinc can be found in dairy products, milk, animal food (like meat) and whole-grain products (52).

If you consume too much of zinc the risk of developing cardiovascular diseases are increased (more than 150 mg of zinc per day), you may get fever and dizziness and your ability to absorb other minerals will be reduced (52).

Recommendations of zinc

The recommended intake of zinc for men is 9 milligrams per day and for women 7 milligrams per day. The lowest recommended intake for men is 5 milligrams per day and for women 4 milligrams per day. The highest recommended intake is not established for both men and women (57).

Iodine

One of the most common nutritional disorders in the world today is deficiency of iodine which causes goiter (enlarged thyroid gland). The prevalence of goiter has decreased due to fortification with iodine in table salt and bread. Iodine in plants occurs mainly in inorganic forms and the content of iodine is higher in sea-plants than in plants grown on land. The content of iodine is usually higher in winter milk than in summer milk. Shellfish, marine fish and eggs contain high concentrations of iodine (60,61). Other sources of iodine are cereals, potatoes, vegetables, mussels and lobster (52).

Iodine from the diet is absorbed as iodide generally efficiently while protein-bound iodine and iodine from seaweed are absorbed in smaller amounts. Around 90 % of the 200 micrograms of iodine from a mixed diet is excreted through the urine. Small amounts are also lost through the feces and the skin. Goitrogens, mainly Sulphur-containing glucosides (glucosinolates) found in Brassica species like Brussels sprouts, cabbage, rapeseeds and turnips inhibit the uptake of iodine into the thyroid gland or causes problems in the production of the hormones (62).

Iodine is responsible for the thyroid hormones T3 and T4 which provide increased glycogenolysis and lipogenolysis. The thyroid hormones are also responsible for increased absorption of glucose, cell metabolism, protein synthesis and ATP (increases the number and size of mitochondria). You can find the most of iodine in the thyroid (around 70 – 80 % of all iodine) (52).

The human body absorbs approximately 90 % of the iodine and it transports to the thyroid gland in the thyroid hormones (52).

If you consume 2 milligrams of iodine per day it can lead to, in rare cases, nasal congestion, rhinitis (inflammation and irritation in the nose's mucous membrane), headache, swollen salivary glands, acne-like skin changes, disturbances in thyroid function like goiter, inflammation in the thyroid gland (auto-immune thyroiditis), and hyper- or hypothyroidism (63).

Deficiency of iodine usually results in non-toxic goiter which means that the thyroid gland is enlarged but the synthesis of the hormones is normal. Non-toxic goiter can develop to toxic goiter which means that the secretion of hormones are increased and the metabolism increases later on (thyrotoxicosis). The thyroid gland can be enlarged either with focal changes (nodular goiter) or in a diffuse form (Graves' disease or Basedow's disease). Severe deficiency of iodine can lead to cretinism which includes mental disturbances, impaired growth, and disturbances in acuity and speech (deaf mutism) in children and infants, and in adults, hypothyroidism (myxedema) can occur (62,64).

According to World Health Organization (WHO), around 1.6 billion people have a higher risk of developing iodine deficiency and around 20 million people have mental defects caused by iodine deficiency (52).

Recommendations of iodine

The recommended intake of iodine for both women and men is 150 micrograms per day. The lowest recommended intake for both women and men is 70 micrograms per day and the highest recommended intake for both women and men is 600 micrograms per day (60).

Selenium

Selenium is found in selenoproteins as selenocysteine and is also found in all tissues as selenomethionine. The thyroid hormone metabolism and co-factor in antioxidant activities are the functions of selenium. Severe deficiency of selenium can lead to cardiomyopathy (diseases that affect the heart muscle) and extreme amounts over the highest recommended intake can lead to toxic symptoms (65).

The inorganic forms of selenium (selenate and selenite) are only found in dietary supplements and not in foods. You can find selenium in eggs, fish and other seafood, offal, meat, dairy products and cereal products. Around 80 % of selenium is absorbed when it comes from dietary sources (65,66,67).

Dietary selenium (mainly organic selenium in forms like selenocysteine and selenomethionine) and water-soluble selenium compounds are absorbed in the body effectively, and organic selenium and selenates are better absorbed than selenites. Compounds of selenium are always converted to selenides before incorporation to selenoproteins. Selenomethionine is converted to selenide before incorporation to proteins. Detoxified excretory products like trimethyl selenonium and dimethyl selenide ions are formed when the intake of selenium is high, but trimethyl selenonium is excreted through the urine and dimethyl selenide is excreted through the lungs.

The human selenoproteome consist of 25 selenoproteins where the following are glutathione peroxidases (GSHPx) include extracellular (eGSHPx), cellular (cGSHPx), gastrointestinal (giGSHPx) and phospholipid hydroperoxide (phGSHPx) and in connection with metalloenzymes, these are good protectors for oxidative damage to the tissues. The activity of the selenoprotein thioedoxin reductases are also affected by selenium. Selenoprotein P functions as an antioxidative protective enzyme and it also functions as transport protein for selenium, and it also might be a good protector against lipid peroxidation to low-density lipoproteins and endothelial cells (67,68).

If you consume enough selenium, the risk of cancer may be reduced (52).

Deficiency of selenium is uncommon in the world except in regions in China. If you consume too little of selenium, it can lead to cardiomyopathy (Keshan disease), myocardial infarction, cardiovascular diseases, osteoarthropathy (metaphyseal involvement with shortened toes and fingers and swollen joints) and myxedema with development of cretinism (68). If you on the other hand consume too much selenium, it can lead to liver damage, vomiting, nausea, garlic-like breath odour, peripheral nerve damage, hair and nail deformities (250 mg of selenium per day) (69).

Recommendations of selenium

The recommended intake for men is 60 micrograms per day and the recommended intake for women is 50 micrograms per day. The lowest recommended intake is 20 micrograms per day for both men and women. The highest recommended intake for both men and women is 300 micrograms per day (65).

Copper

Copper is responsible for the reduction and oxidation processes inside cells, electron transport chain, iron and energy metabolism and protects against free radicals, the formation of connective tissues. You can find the most copper in the liver in the body. Copper is transported to the liver via albumin, plasma and amino acids in the blood (52).

There is high concentrations of copper in offal and liver, low concentrations of copper in milk products and milk, and intermediate concentrations of copper in chocolate products, meats, grain products, tomatoes, mushrooms, dried fruits, potatoes and bananas (70).

Copper is absorbed to 35 % - 70 % in the small intestine when the intake of copper is between 1 – 5 milligrams per day. If you consume more copper, the absorption will decrease, and if you consume less copper, the absorption will increase. Copper is either chelated by metallothionein (is induced by zinc and prevents copper to be transported into the blood circulation) or is bound to a copper chaperone in the enterocytes in the small intestine. If you consume 50 milligrams per day of zinc, the absorption of copper will be inhibited. When copper will be absorbed in the blood circulation, the copper chaperones transport the copper to proteins that transport copper into the blood circulation. When the copper has been absorbed in the blood circulation, copper binds to transcuprein, complexes of low molecular weight copper histidine, albumin or a combination of all these and is then transported to the liver, where it binds to either reduced glutathione or metallothionein and is stored in the cells. In the plasma, most of the copper is transported as ceruloplasmin which the liver produces. The copper is lost through the bile and urine.

In the body of an adult person, there is between 50 – 120 milligrams of copper and there is around 6 % copper in erythrocytes and plasma, 10 % in the brain, 15 % in the liver, and 40 % in muscle tissue.

Symptoms of deficiency of copper is anemia, low concentrations of white blood cells, skin- and hair depigmentation, skeletal- and heart abnormalities, cardiac- and immune dysfunction, increased risk of cancer in the colorectum (due to increased production of faecel free radicals, increased cytotoxicity and increased faecal water alkaline phosphatase activity).

If you consume too much of copper it can lead to nausea, gastric pain, diarrhea, vomiting and increased risk of childhood sclerosis when storage of food are in non-galvanized copper containers.

In areas where there is soft water, copper from copper tubes can leach out and cause gastrointestinal disorders due to high concentrations of copper, and therefore, a good recommendation is that the tap water should run for some seconds before consumption (70,71,72,73,74).

There is a disease called Menke's syndrome which is genetic and means that the person has a decreased absorption of copper and has a mental retardation. Another disease called Wilson's syndrome means that the person has neurological problems and liver accumulation. These diseases affect copper in a bad way (52).

Recommendations of copper

The recommended intake for adults is 0.9 milligrams per day. The lowest recommended intake for adults is 0.4 milligrams per day and the highest recommended intake for adults is 5.0 milligrams per day (70).

Chromium

In foods and dietary supplements, trivalent chromium (III) which is an ionic form of chromium is the most common in there. Trivalent chromium (III) is ubiquitous in nature and is found in the water, air, biological materials and soil. Dichromates and chromates are formed by hexavalent chromium (IV) and these can traverse biological membranes and are strong oxidizers. Hexavalent chromium are mutagenic, toxic and environmental contaminants, and they rarely occur in the environment (75).

You can find chromium in pulses, nuts, fish, spices, whole grain products and processed meats (75).

The absorption of trivalent chromium is around 0.4 – 2.5 % in the body and the rest is excreted through sweat, urine and the bile. Organic chromium compounds have a more efficient absorption, but as soon as they are absorbed, the compounds will be excreted through the bile rapidly. It has been proven that the absorption of chromium increases when ascorbate is administered simultaneous and when there is deficiency of iron and zinc in the body.

Deficiency symptoms of chromium in humans are weight loss, impaired glucose tolerance and glucose utilization, increased plasma fatty acids concentrations, neuropathy, abnormalities in nitrogen metabolism and depressed respiratory quotient. After 200 micrograms per day of chromium supplementation, the symptoms improved. Chromium has been suggested to be important for lipid, carbohydrate and protein metabolism through chromium's effect on insulin action, and therefore, chromium has also been suggested to be a cofactor for insulin (76).

High intakes of trivalent chromium (III) around 1 – 2 grams per day have not been associated with negative health effects. On the other hand, chromium picolinate (a trivalent chromium compound that is common in many food supplements) might cause negative health effects on the central nervous system (the behavior will be affected), kidneys and potential clastogenicity. The UK Food Standards Agency gives the advice to people to not consume chromium picolinate because it can cause cancer (77).

Recommendations of chromium

There are no recommendations of chromium in the Nordic countries due to lack of sufficient evidence, but in, for example, Australia and New Zealand, the recommended intake of chromium is 35 micrograms per day for men and 25 micrograms per day for women. The US Food and Nutrition Board has the same recommendations of adequate intake of chromium on adults between 19 and 50 years (78). When it comes to chromium, the best option for you, is to check the recommended intake of chromium in your country, so you don't consume too much or too little of it.

Manganese

Manganese is important for the activation of enzymes that are participated in the production of mucopolysaccharides, proteins and cholesterol. Manganese works also as a catalytic cofactor for pyruvate carboxylase, arginase and mitochondrial superoxide dismutase.

Tea, nuts, wholegrain cereals and leafy vegetables contain high concentrations of manganese (79).

In the body, we have around 10 – 20 milligrams of manganese and high concentrations are found in bone, in organs rich in mitochondria like the pancreas, liver and kidney. There are low concentrations of manganese in plasma and muscle. Around 5 % of manganese is absorbed in the body through the diet, and through the bile are the most manganese lost. In humans, it has been shown that the absorption of manganese is negatively affected by calcium, and the absorption of iron is inhibited by high intakes of manganese, and there has also been shown that the absorption of manganese increases when there is deficiency of iron (79,80).

Manganese toxicity have been found in workers in manganese mines and these persons have been observed to have neurological- and psychological changes like Parkinson's disease (a long-term degenerative disorder that affects the motor system in the central nervous system). The nervous system of children may be negatively affected by manganese from drinking water (81).

Deficiency symptoms of manganese are hypercholesterolemia (too high levels of cholesterol in the blood), dermal changes, diffuse bone demineralization and reduced growth in children (80).

Recommendations of manganese

There are no recommendations of manganese in the Nordic countries due to lack of sufficient evidence, but in Australia and New Zealand, the recommended intake of manganese is 5.5 milligrams per day for men in the age of 19 – 70+ years old and for women in the age of 19 – 70+ years old 5 milligrams per day. The EU Scientific Committee for Food suggested that an acceptable intake of manganese would be between 1 – 10 milligrams per day, in 1993. The US Total Diet Study 1982 – 1989 set an adequate intake for adult women to be 1.8 milligrams per day and for adult men to be 2.3 milligrams per day (80).

Molybdenum

There are three molybdenum-containing enzymes known in humans which are xanthine oxidase, sulphite oxidase and aldehyde oxidase which are important for catabolism of heterocyclic compounds and sulphur-containing amino acids, inclusive pyridines and purines.

Molybdenum exists in the form of soluble molybdates in water and food. The concentration of molybdenum in plants varies very much due to pH and concentration of molybdenum in the soil. Good food sources of molybdenum are legumes, offal, grains, nuts, eggs and dairy products. Shellfish contains high concentrations of molybdenum. Muscle meat, root vegetables and fruits contain low concentrations of molybdenum (82).

Around 80 % of molybdenum is absorbed in the body and the content of molybdenum is regulated by the kidneys. Molybdenum deficiency has been observed in one human with Chrohn's disease. The symptoms of deficiency of molybdenum include heart disturbances, unconsciousness, and night blindness, but these symptoms disappeared when the human received 160 micrograms per day of supplementation with molybdenum (83).

Recommendations of molybdenum

There are no recommendations of molybdenum in the Nordic countries due to lack of sufficient evidence, but in Australia and New Zealand, the recommended intake of molybdenum is 45 micrograms per day for both women and men in the age of 19 – 70+ years old. Even The US Food and Nutrition Board have set the same intake of 45 micrograms molybdenum per day for adult women and men (83). The highest recommended intake of molybdenum is 2 milligrams per day, according to The US Food and Nutrition Board, and according to The Scientific Committee on Food, the highest recommended intake of molybdenum is 0.6 milligrams per day for adults (84).

Fluoride

Fluoride bound to complexes or in an ionic form is found in drinking water and food. Fluoride helps to treat and prevent dental caries. The highest concentrations of fluoride are found in some teas, canned sardines, drinking water in some areas and some mineral waters (85).

90 % of the fluoride in drinking water is absorbed in the body, but fluoride that is complex-bound is not so good absorbed in the body. Through the kidneys, around 50 % of the total absorbed fluoride is excreted and the rest of the fluoride is integrated in bones and teeth (children) (86). Flour helps to inhibit bacterial enzymes and is resistant to acid erosion. You can find flour in some toothpastes (52).

In adults, 2.2 grams/kg bodyweight of fluoride intake is lethal. 5 milligrams per kg bodyweight leads to stomach pain, nausea and vomiting. Chronic high intakes might damage kidney function and skeletal mineralization, and the common side effect is enamel fluorosis which consists of a sub-surface enamel that is hypomineralized and above this layer is enamel that is well-mineralized. Thyroid metabolism has also been affected by a high intake of fluoride, but not from fluoride in drinking water or in toothpastes (86,87).

Recommendations of fluoride

There are no recommendations of fluoride in the Nordic countries due to lack of sufficient evidence, but in Australia and New Zealand, the recommended intake of fluoride is 4 milligrams per day for men between the age 19 – 70+ years and 3 milligrams per day for women in the age between 19 – 70+ years. The US Institute of Medicine also set the adequate intake of 4 milligrams per day for men and 3 milligrams per day for women (22, Page 622). The EFSA (European Food Safety Authority) set the highest recommended intake of fluoride to be 7 milligrams per day for adults (22, Page 623).

Now I have described some minerals that are important for the body. There are a few more minerals that exist but I chose to describe the most important. Now I will describe the fat-soluble vitamins that are important for the body.

Let's start with the definition of a vitamin. A vitamin is available in food, is an organic substance, is synthetic, is essential, is available in small quantities, has different functions in the body depending on which vitamin it is, when we don't have enough of a vitamin in our body we will get injured. The vitamins cannot be produced by the human being, therefore we need to consume them from the food (52).

Vitamin A

Vitamin A can be in the form of preformed vitamin A in the diet as either Retinol and its fatty acyl esters mainly found in fish liver oils and animal sources like eggs, milk, butter and in many mono- and multivitamin supplements or as provitamin A carotenoids mainly found in orange or red-coloured vegetables and fruits and in dark-green leafy vegetables (88). Retinol and Retinyl ester are to 70 – 90 % absorbed in the body while provitamin A carotenoids are absorbed to 5 – 60 %, but if you add some extra fat like vegetable oil you can increase the absorption of Carotene (89).

Carotenoids such as beta-cryptoxanthin and alpha- and beta-carotene are absorbed in the body through passive diffusion. After the passive diffusion, the provitamin A carotenoids enter the enterocytes and are being cleaved and produces one or two molecules of retinol. Before the retinyl esters can enter the enterocytes they must go through an enzymatic conversion to retinol in the intestinal lumen. 70 – 90 % of retinol enters then the chylomicrons esterified with long-chain fatty acids and can then be absorbed. The most of the chylomicron retinyl esters are then being transported to the liver. In the hepatic stellate cells, approximately 50 % - 80 % of the body's total retinol is stored as retinyl esters for several months.

To ensure supply of retinol to target cells, retinol bound to retinol-binding protein is released from the liver and is looking for retinol in the plasma in the blood. When the retinol is in the target cells, it is oxidized to retinoic acid and retinal (the active metabolites of retinol) and these metabolites are often produced in these cells. Retinoic acid is responsible for the activation of nuclear retinoic acid receptors which modulates gene transcription and the retinal is related to the visual process as a chromophore (90,91).

Vitamin A is responsible for the eyesight, gene transcription, epithelial differentiation, reproduction, transport, bone metabolism, growth development and immune competence (89).

If you consume too little of vitamin A, it can lead to dry eyes, night blindness, blindness, impaired resistance to infection, nails that cracks, dry skin, dry hairs, infertility, skin irritation and loss of appetite (89).
If you consume too much of Vitamin A, it can lead to irritation, headache, tiredness, dizziness, reduced bone mineral density, embryonic malformations, increased risk for hip fracture, cellular toxicity in the liver, and

eventually cirrhosis and fibrosis in the liver and hepatotoxicity. If you consume too much of Carotenoids (like carrots) you can become orange, but it is not dangerous for you (89).

You can find Vitamin A as retinol in liver, low-fat milk, edible fat, spinach, dairy products, margarine and spreads. Vitamin A as carotenoids, you can mainly find in beta-carotene plant products like orange or red-colored vegetables and fruits and in dark-green leafy vegetables (88).

Recommendations of Vitamin A

The recommended intake for women is 700 micrograms per day and the lowest recommended intake is 400 micrograms per day and the highest recommended intake is 3000 micrograms (3 grams) per day.

The recommended intake for men is 900 micrograms per day and the lowest recommended intake is 500 micrograms per day and the highest recommended intake is 3000 micrograms per day. These recommendations on vitamin A include both some provitamin A carotenoids and vitamin A as retinol, and a term called 'retinol equivalents' (RE) is used as recommendations in the diet, therefore, for example, 900 micrograms per day of vitamin A for men has to come both from provitamin A carotenoids and vitamin A as retinol (92,88).

Vitamin D

Vitamin D is in the form of cholecalciferol D_3 and is mainly found in some animal foods and the basic requirements of vitamin D_3 can be satisfied through the sunlight (93) and ergocalciferol D_2 mainly found in mushrooms. Vitamin D and cholesterol are very similar to each other. You can find Vitamin D in the liver in the body. When the Vitamin D is stored in the liver it is called 25 (OH) D_2 and in the kidneys it is called 25 (OH) D_3 (32). Naturally vitamin D is absorbed in the small intestine in the body via the lymphatic system incorporated in chylomicrons. Around 80 % of the vitamin D is absorbed through this way (94).

The liver is the organ that takes up vitamin D_3 from the gut or produced in the skin. In the liver, vitamin D_3 is hydroxylated to 25OHD, which is a metabolite that is bound to the vitamin D binding protein in plasma where it is transported. 25OHD is transported to the kidneys where it is converted to calcitriol (1,25-dihydroxyvitamin D) which is a hormone that regulates the calcium and phosphate levels in the plasma together with calcitonin and parathyroid hormone when it is bound to a nuclear vitamin D receptor. Calcitriol's mainly function is to ensure that calcium is being absorbed from the intestine. Calcitriol together with parathyroid hormone release calcium from the bone, so that the concentrations of calcium in the plasma is increasing (95).

Vitamin D is important for the skeleton, teeth, kidneys, normal mineralization of the skeleton, the immune system, cell proliferation and differentiation, calcium homeostasis, regulating calcium uptake in the body's cells and secreting insulin. It is also important for thyroid and thyroid hormones (89).

If you consume too little of Vitamin D it can lead to the metabolic syndrome because fat cells have receptors for Vitamin D, rickets in children and infants, osteomalacia in adults, osteopenia (not enough of calcium to the bone tissues) and soft bones.

Older people produces less Vitamin D than younger people, therefore older people need more Vitamin D than the younger people (89).

If you consume too much of Vitamin D it can lead to calcification. This can lead to cardiovascular disease problems if vascular muscles and vascular walls are calcified (89). Too much of vitamin D can also lead to gastrointestinal symptoms, increased risk of mortality, increased risk of prostate cancer and total cancer (96).

You can find Vitamin D mainly in edible fats, oily fish, milk products, margarine, chanterelles, egg yolk and oils. You can find vitamin D_3 in lean freshwater fish, eggs and meat. You can also get Vitamin D from the sunlight. 7-Dehydrocholesterol → (Provitamin D) UV light → (Previtamin D) Heat → Vitamin D_3. That is how the sunlight turns into Vitamin D_3 in the body.

You can also get Vitamin D from the breast milk, but children need more Vitamin D in form of supplement, because the breast milk does not consist enough of Vitamin D (89).

Recommendations of Vitamin D

The recommended intake of vitamin D for men and women is 10 micrograms per day in the Nordic countries. The lowest recommended intake of vitamin D is 2.5 micrograms per day and the highest recommended intake of vitamin D is 100 micrograms per day (93).

People in the Nordic countries like Sweden, Norway, Finland, Denmark and Iceland need more vitamin D in the wintertime than people in countries where the sun is shining more in the wintertime like Australia and USA. Therefore, you MUST look up what the recommended intake of vitamin D is in your country, because the recommendations vary a lot between some countries. For example, in Sweden, the recommended intake is 10 micrograms per day for both men and women and in Australia and New Zealand the recommended intake for men and women between the age 19 – 50 years old is 5 micrograms per day and for men and women between the age 51 – 70 years old 10 micrograms per day. So, it is very important that you check the recommendations of vitamin D in just your country, because the sun has different effect in different countries.

At latitudes around 60 degrees north during the summer months (June and July), exposure of the arms, face and hands (25 % of body surface) to the sun for six to eight minutes two or three times per week provides 5 – 10 micrograms of Vitamin D3 per day in individuals with fair skin pigmentation and approximately 10 – 15 minutes per day is required for individuals with darker pigmentation (97,94).

Vitamin E

The most of the Vitamin E has its end destination in the liver and the bile (can be reabsorbed when it goes back to the intestine). Around 20 – 40 % of the Vitamin E is absorbed in the body. Vitamin E is transported with LDL, HDL or VLDL to tissues that are in need of Vitamin E.

The vitamin is transported in the form of an antioxidant or a vitamin.

Vitamin E has four forms which are alpha, beta, gamma and delta where alpha has the highest vitamin activity but the lowest antioxidant capacity (89).

The absorption of vitamin E requires presence of pancreatic enzymes, bile salts and the formation of micelles. When the vitamin E is absorbed, it is transported bound to HDL in the liver where alpha-tocopherol is bound to alpha-tocopherol transport protein which is important for the resecretion of alpha-tocopherol. The absorbed vitamin E can also be transported within chylomicrons. Sometimes, some alpha-tocopherol is not released into the circulation and this alpha-tocopherol is instead excreted to the bile via transporters or is metabolized through a cytochrome called cytochrome P450 system. The alpha-tocopherol is excreted mainly through feces and small amounts through urine. It takes decades to get rid of vitamin E in the body when it has been absorbed. Alpha-tocopherol is the common tocopherol in human tissues where it contributes around 90 % of the total amount of tocotrienols and tocopherols in plasma and 50 – 80 % in other tissues. It has been showed that a high intake of vitamin E can result in prolonged bleeding because the vitamin E might interfere with the blood clotting system especially when vitamin E is consumed together with anticoagulants or aspirin (98,99,100).

You can find Vitamin E in cell membranes where it protects our membranes and plasma lipoproteins from propagation of free radicals (99).

The Vitamin E (alpha-tocopherol) is responsible for antioxidant activity, inactive different enzymes, the protection of lipoproteins and cell membranes, cellular signaling, cell development, gene expression, our cells in the vessels. If you consume enough of Vitamin E, cardiovascular diseases are counteracted (89). Supplementations of alpha-tocopherol have not been proven to decrease oxidative stress (100).

If you have lost Vitamin E, you can start the production again by consuming ascorbic acid (Vitamin C) (89).

If you consume too little of Vitamin E it can lead to impaired immune function, deteriorated reproduction, hemolytic anemia and neuropathy (101).

You can find a lot of Vitamin E in vegetable oil-based spreads, vegetable oils, seeds, nuts, egg yolk, cereal products, fish and shellfish. If you want the highest content of alpha-tocopherol then you will use sunflower oil, but it is also a lot of alpha-tocopherol in corn and rapeseed oil and olive oil and soybean oil (98).

Recommendations of vitamin E
The recommended intake of vitamin E is 8 milligrams per day for women and 10 milligrams per day for men. The lowest recommended intake is 3 milligrams per day for women and 4 milligrams per day for men and the highest recommended intake is 300 milligrams per day for both men and women (101).

Vitamin K

Vitamin K is a collective term for compounds that have vitamin K activity and all these compounds have the same structure in common, which is the 2-methyl-1,4-naphtoquinone ring structure. Vitamin K can be in two forms, either vitamin K_1 (Phylloquinone) with the structure (2-methyl-3-phytyl-1,4-naphtoquinone) or vitamin K_2 (Menaquinones) with the structure (multi-isoprenylquinones, several species). Vitamin K_1 is produced by plants and vitamin K_2 is produced by bacteria. Both vitamins are found in tissues in animals (102).

You can find vitamin K_1 mainly in vegetable oils, leafy green vegetables and vegetable oil based fat spreads. Vitamin K_2 is mainly found in egg yolk, meat, liver and dairy products (102).

In the ileum and jejunum, vitamin K is absorbed and around 80 % is absorbed of purified vitamin K_1. From food sources, vitamin K_1 is absorbed to approximately 10

– 15 %. Bleeding and fat malabsorption (less uptake of fat in the diet) decrease the absorption of vitamin K. Absorbed vitamin K is mainly taken up by the liver and is transported in the lymph in chylomicrons to the liver. Vitamin K is also stored in the pancreas, the heart, the bone tissue and the fat tissue. To maintain satisfactory body stores, vitamin K is required to be consumed due to the hepatic reserves are rapidly depleted when insufficient vitamin K is consumed in the diet (103).

Vitamin K is responsible for building in calcium in the legs and producing thrombin and prothrombin together with the calcium metabolism (89).

If you consume too little of Vitamin K it can lead to skeletal problems (interaction with calcium). Older people can produce less Vitamin K which can lead to diseases (89).

The people that may need extra Vitamin K is newborns because they have a lower placenta transport and people who have malabsorption (lower absorption), use antibiotics and parental nutrition without vitamin K supplementation (104).

Recommendations of vitamin K

There are different recommendations in different countries of vitamin K. For example, in the Nordic countries, there are no recommendation of vitamin K due to lack of sufficient evidence while in USA the recommended intake is 90 micrograms per day for women, 120 micrograms per day for men and in Australia and New Zealand, the recommended intake is 70 micrograms per day for men and 60 micrograms per day for women (89). You must check the recommendations in your country to ensure that you get enough of vitamin K.

The following nine vitamins that I will describe are called water-soluble vitamins. These vitamins are absorbed in jejunum except for the vitamin B12 which is absorbed in the terminal ileum. The water-soluble vitamins are transported freely or protein bounded in the blood. These

vitamins are stored in muscles or liver and some vitamins
are stored in all cells. We lose the water-soluble vitamins
from the urine (kidneys).

The first water-soluble vitamin I will describe is Vitamin
C.

Vitamin C

Vitamin C is a term for dehydroascorbic acid and
ascorbic acid because these both forms have an effect that
is anti-scorbutic. You can find vitamin C in many berries,
vegetables and fruits like blackcurrants, orange,
clementine and kiwi (105).

Vitamin C is a cofactor for many enzymes that are
involved in the biosynthesis of carnitine,
neurotransmitters and collagen. When it comes to these
effects, ascorbic acid works as an electron donor. In the
body, ascorbic acid will be oxidized to dehydroascorbic
acid. Vitamin C is also responsible for the biosynthesis of
aldosterone, corticosteroids and in the conversion of

cholesterol to bile acids through microsomal hydroxylation of cholesterol. The absorption of non-heme iron is improved by ascorbic acid due to its reducing power. Ascorbic acid can also inactivate nitrosamines which are carcinogenic substances and it can also protect semen, neutrophils and plasma against LDL-oxidation. The bioavailability of vitamin C is most effective for doses of 100 milligrams or less, where the bioavailability is at least 80 %. Doses of 200 – 500 milligrams, the bioavailability decreases to 60 – 70 %, and doses over 500 to 1000 milligrams, the bioavailability is less than 50 %. Vitamin C that is not absorbed due to too large doses of vitamin C is degraded in the intestine and this can result in intestinal discomfort and diarrhea. The transport protein of vitamin C can only be filled with a certain amount of vitamin C, and when this transport protein is filled, the remaining vitamin C will be excreted in the urine. Doses of 60 milligrams or less result in no excretion of vitamin C. For doses of 100 milligrams, around ¼ is excreted, for doses of 200 milligrams, around ½ is excreted and for doses of 500 milligrams, around 80 – 90 % is excreted. At around 100 milligrams, the body pool of ascorbic acid is filled up and at this concentration, monocytes, neutrophils and lymphocytes become saturated (106,107).

Vitamin C is responsible for the production of collagen, bones and skin (consists of collagen), the electron transport, vitamin C works as a redox system, it has an antioxidant function, it is an enzyme co-substrate, it is also a catecholamine, transmitter, peptide hormone and it is responsible for the production of catecholamine (108).

Vitamin C is very healthy for our body and therefore it has health effects. It helps us to reduce inflammation, reduce the risk of cardiovascular diseases (the LDL oxidation decreases), reduce high stress, reduce the risk of diabetes, cataract (the eyes) and cancer. Vitamin C helps to improve the immune function, it helps to improve the skin, teeth, pregnancy and the lung function (108). It has been proven that supplementation of around 200 – 1000 milligrams of vitamin C might reduce the common cold's duration with around 10 % (109).

You can find Vitamin C in the kidneys, spinal fluid, muscles, brain, plasma, liver, the eye and in red blood cells. The vitamin C can stay in the body for 60 – 100 days. If you consume too much vitamin C, the absorption decreases (108).

If you don't consume enough Vitamin C, it can lead to skin problems, muscle weakness, infections, hemorrhoids and bleeding.
If you on the other hand, consume too much of Vitamin C, it can lead to dizziness, stomach ache, diarrhea and kidney stones.
Breastfeeding women and pregnant women should consume more Vitamin C (108).

Vitamin E can be beneficially for the uptake of Vitamin C (108).

Recommendations of vitamin C
The recommended intake of vitamin C for both men and women is 75 milligrams per day. The lowest recommended intake for both men and women is 10

milligrams per day. There is no highest recommended intake established (105).

Vitamin B$_1$ (Thiamin)

Vitamin B$_1$ or Thiamin, which it also can be called, is important for the utilization of branched-chain amino acids and carbohydrates in the body (110). It works like a vitamin K. In the blood, Vitamin B$_1$, is transported with a protein called thiamin-binding protein. You can find Vitamin B$_1$ in the heart, muscles, brain, liver and kidneys. We lose the vitamin through the urine.

Vitamin B$_1$ can stay in the body for 9 – 18 days which means that we must regularly consume the vitamin or else it can lead to heart muscle problems, neural problems, weight loss that is not healthy and anorexia (108).

Thiamin is occurred in phosphorylated forms in animal foods which are being converted into free thiamin when it is absorbed in the body. Thiamin is occurred in free forms in vegetable forms. In the small intestine, thiamin is absorbed through an active, carrier-mediated system which involves phosphorylation, but if the intake of thiamin is high, then passive diffusion is also involved in the absorption process. Thiamin is also obtained in the large intestine's bacterial flora where it also is absorbed. Around 95 % of thiamin is absorbed in the body. Right after the absorption, thiamin is transported in the blood to the liver. In the liver, thiamin is converted to thiamin pyrophosphate, its biologically active form (111).

If you don't consume enough of vitamin B_1, it can lead to neural dysfunction (Dry Beri Beri), heart muscle problems (edema, Wet Beri Beri), infantile Beri Beri (if the mother has a lack of vitamin B_1 when she is breastfeeding) and Wernicke's encephalopathy and Korsakoff's psychosis syndrome that is usually common in people who drink way too much alcohol (108).

You can find Vitamin B_1 in whole grain cereal, cereals, meat, milk, dairy products, beans and pork.

If you consume raw fish, seafood, coffee or tea, the absorption will be destroyed due to thiaminas and phenols in the food (108).

Recommendations of vitamin B$_1$ (Thiamin)

The recommended intake for men is 1.4 milligrams per day and for women it is 1.1 milligrams per day. The lowest recommended intake is 0.6 milligrams per day for men and 0.5 milligrams per day for women. The highest recommended intake for men and women is not established (110).

Vitamin B$_2$ (Riboflavin)

In foods, Riboflavin or Vitamin B$_2$, which it also can be called, occurs as flavin mononucleotide or flavin adenine dinucleotide complexed with proteins or as a free molecule. In the gastrointestinal tract, protein-bound riboflavin is converted (hydrolyzed) to free riboflavin. The absorption rates of riboflavin is between 50 – 60 % for free riboflavin and 60 – 70 % of riboflavin in whole foods. In the body, riboflavin is mainly stored as flavoproteins and a smaller amount of free riboflavin. The urinary excretion of riboflavin can be increased during infections or during negative nitrogen balance. The urinary excretion of riboflavin can, instead, be decreased during rapid growth (112,113).

Vitamin B_2 is responsible for the carbohydrate metabolism, lipid metabolism, amino acid metabolism, energy metabolism, the skin health (33) and the folate metabolism because Flavin adenine dinucleotide is a co-enzyme for MTHFR (Methylenetetrahydrofolate reductase) which is responsible for homocysteine's metabolism (113).

Vitamin B_2 is very healthy and therefore it has some health effects. Vitamin B_2 helps to reduce the risk of vascular disease, oxidative stress (protects cells and red blood cells), improves the lipid metabolism. Vitamin B2 helps to improve the absorption of zinc ions and iron ions (108).

If you don't consume enough of Vitamin B_2, it can lead to skin changes like cheilosis and glossitis (has to do with the tongue), inflammation, hypersensitivity in the eye, anemia, neuropathy.

If you consume a high intake of protein, you must increase the intake of Vitamin B_2.

It is, on the other hand, very hard to overdose Vitamin B_2 (108).

You can find Vitamin B_2 in animal products, cheese, milk (the best source), fermented milk products and legumes (108).

Recommendations of vitamin B_2 (Riboflavin)

The recommended intake for men is 1.7 milligrams per day and for women 1.3 milligrams per day. The lowest recommended intake of riboflavin is 0.8 milligrams per day for both men and women. The highest recommended intake for men and women is not established (112).

Vitamin B_3 (Niacin)

Niacin is a term for nicotinamide, nicotinic acid, and derivatives that exhibit nicotinamide's biological activity.

Niacin is very responsible for many redox reactions in the metabolism of amino acids, glucose and fatty acids in the form of NAD (nicotinamide adenine dinucleotide) or/and NADP (nicotinamide adenine dinucleotide phosphate) (114).

NAD and NADP are the forms which niacin occurs in foods, and these forms are absorbed and hydrolyzed in the intestine. The nicotinic acid is absorbed up to almost 3 grams. If the niacin is esterified to polysaccharides, which happens when niacin occurs in cereals like maize, this form is less available for the body. The amino acid tryptophan can be converted to niacin, where 60 mg tryptophan gives 1 mg of niacin, which is not that effective (114,115).

Niacin is responsible for the skin health, gastrointestinal tract, nervous system and energy metabolism. When you consume niacin, you must consume vitamin B_1, B_2 and B_6 (108). Niacin can stay in the body for up to 50 - 60 days after it is absorbed, then deficiency symptoms can occur (115).

If you don't consume enough of niacin, it can lead to shortness of breath (pellagra), inflamed skin (dermatitis), dementia, diarrhea and even death (108). If you consume too much of niacin, the results might be flushing and liver damage (116).

In fish, meat and pulses, you can find niacin in the form of preformed niacin and in protein-rich foods you can find niacin converted from tryptophan (114).

Recommendations of vitamin B$_3$ (Niacin)
The recommended intake of niacin for men is 18 milligrams per day and 15 milligrams per day for women. The lowest recommended intake per day is 12 milligrams for men and 9 milligrams for women. The highest recommended intake per day is 35 milligrams for both men and women (114).

Vitamin B₅ (Pantothenic acid)

Pantothenic acid is water-soluble and is a vitamin in the group of B-vitamins. Pantothenic acid is participated in the intermediary metabolism as part of coenzyme A. You can find pantothenic acid in cheese, milk, vegetables, meats, cereal products (including bread), dried legumes, offal and wholegrain products. The best sources are dried legumes, offal and wholegrain products (117).

Pantothenic acid is important for anabolism and catabolism as a carrier of acyl groups. Around 40 – 60 % of the vitamin is absorbed in the body. Deficiency of pantothenic acid is very rare and very few people have had deficiency. The people who have had deficiency symptoms have not eaten enough of pantothenic acid in their diets or has been given an antagonist to pantothenic acid.

Some people believe that the humans' hair color can be restored by the help of pantothenic acid, but this is not true (117).

Vitamin B5 is also responsible for hemoglobin, hormones, lipids and the energy metabolism (108).

Recommendations of pantothenic acid

There is no recommended intake of pantothenic acid in the Nordic countries due to lack of sufficient evidence. In the US, the recommended intake of pantothenic acid is 5 milligrams per day for adults (118). In New Zealand and Australia, the recommended intake for men is 6 milligrams per day and for women 4 milligrams per day.

Vitamin B6

Vitamin B6 is a term for pyridoxal, pyridoxine and pyridoxamine (119). Vitamin B6 is responsible for the glycogen metabolism, amino acid metabolism and cognitive and immune functions. In the blood, vitamin B6 is transported with plasma proteins to the tissues. Vitamin B6 can be absorbed in the body very easily (108).

In the gut via a passive process, the absorption of the different vitamers of vitamin B6 takes place. Pyridoxine raises the concentrations of pyridoxal phosphate 10 % more than pyridoxamine and pyridoxal.

Around 170 milligrams of vitamin B_6 is stored in the body, where 80 – 90 % of this content is found in the muscles. Vitamin B_6 can even be found in the heart, liver and kidneys. After 25 – 33 days, pyridoxal phosphate in plasma are half full, which means that the vitamin excretes relatively fast. 70 – 90 % of vitamin B_6 in plasma are pyridoxal phosphate and this percent level is also for the stores in tissues and for the intake of vitamin B_6. The levels of pyridoxal phosphate can also be affected by physical activity and age.

If you consume a high intake of protein (1.5 grams / kg body weight), the levels of pyridoxal phosphate might decrease with up to 40 %, therefore, you may need to consume extra vitamin B_6 if you consume a high intake of protein. If you have a severe deficiency of vitamin B_2 (riboflavin) it can affect the levels of pyridoxal phosphate (120,121).

You need extra vitamin B6 if you drink large amounts of alcohol or if you are taking pills that contain a high intake of estrogen.

If you don't consume enough of vitamin B6, it can lead to muscular problems, neural problems, vascular problems, coronary heart disease, colorectal cancer, skeletal problems, skin problems and a deteriorated reproduction. Vitamin B6 can be stored in the muscles in very high concentrations which is very dangerous and toxic so be careful of vitamin B6 so you don't consume too much of it, especially supplements that contain vitamin B6 (108). If you, on the other hand, consume too much of vitamin B6, consequences like minor neurological symptoms (50 mg/day or more) and neurotoxicity (500 mg/day or more) can be developed (122).

You can find vitamin B6 in whole grains, animal products, cereals, meat, fish, potatoes, bananas, milk and offal (108).

Recommendations of vitamin B$_6$

The recommended intake per day for men is 1.5 milligrams and for women 1.2 milligrams. The lowest recommended intake for men is 1.0 milligrams per day and for women 0.8 milligrams per day. The highest recommended intake for both men and women is 25 milligrams per day (119).

Biotin

Biotin is a heterocyclic compound that is water-soluble and is a group of the B-vitamins. You can find biotin in wheat bran, egg yolks, rolled oats and offal meats like kidney and liver.

Biotin bound to a protein is digested in the gut and when biotin is absorbed, the enzyme biotinidase must cleave the covalent bond between the protein and the biotin. Half of the biotin in foods can at least be absorbed in the body (123).

Biotin is responsible for the production of fat, the conversion of pyruvate to oxaloacetate (an intermediate in the citric acid cycle), degradation of amino acids, gluconeogenesis, energy metabolism and the production of acetyl-CoA (108). Biotin participants also in carboxylation reactions where it functions as a cofactor (124).

Deficiency of biotin is extremely rare, but if you consume 10 raw egg whites in a day, it can lead to a shortage of biotin because of the antivitamin avidin (glycoprotein) (108). Avidin prevents absorption of biotin, but if you cook the egg, then avidin can't bind to biotin, and the biotin can be absorbed in the body (123).

Recommendations of biotin

In the Nordic countries, there is no recommended intake due to lack of sufficient evidence, but in New Zealand and in Australia, the recommended intake is 30 micrograms per day for men and 25 micrograms per day for women. In USA, the recommended intake for biotin is 30 micrograms per day for both men and women (124). Therefore, the aim of sufficient biotin might be around 25 – 30 micrograms per day for healthy individuals.

Vitamin B$_9$ (Folate)

Folate is a term for compounds that include folic acid and derivatives that have similar nutritional properties as folic acid. Folate can also be called folacin. Folic acid (pteroylmonoglutamic acid, PGA) is built up by three parts, a p-aminobenzoic acid, pteridine ring and glutamic acid. Folic acid cannot be found naturally in foods because it is the synthetic form of folate (found in supplements). In foods, folate consists of pteroylpolyglutamates (contain one to six additional glutamate units).

High concentrations of folate are found in green vegetables, liver and legumes. You can also find folate in vegetables, cereal products (including bread), fruits, dairy products and berries.

The bioavailability of folates is estimated to be around 50 %, but this is a rough estimate. The bioavailability of folates from a diet rich in vegetables, fruit and liver products is estimated to be 80 % (125,126,127).

Before the folates from the foods can be absorbed in jejunum, the folate must be hydrolyzed to monoglutamates by brush border folate conjugase (126). In the jejunum, around 40 – 90 % of the vitamin can be absorbed. Folate is transported with a protein called Plasma Folate Binder Protein. The vitamin can be found in the liver where it can stay for weeks to months. The body loses folate through the kidneys (urine) (108).

Folate is responsible for the same functions as vitamin B_{12} inclusive the amino acid metabolism. Folate is also very healthy and it has some important and beneficially health functions that are beneficial to our body. For example, it protects against cardiovascular diseases, anemia and colorectal cancer. It is also very good against dementia and cognitive functions, but it is also important when it comes to cell replication (108).
The people that are in risk of folate deficiency is young women (primarily), pregnant women (cell division) and alcoholics.
The intake of folate is increased by germination, fermentation and production of cheese while it on the

other hand is reduced by frying, baking, UHT treatment
and pasteurization (108).

Recommendations of vitamin B$_9$ (folate)

The recommended intake of folate is 300 micrograms per
day for men and 300 micrograms per day for women
(400 micrograms per day for women of reproductive
age). The lowest recommended intake of folate is 100
micrograms per day for both men and women. The
highest recommended intake for men and women is not
established (125).

The Scientific Committee on Food recommends 1000
micrograms (1 gram) per day for adults as the highest
recommended intake (128).

Vitamin B$_{12}$ (Cobalamin)

Vitamin B$_{12}$ is a term for corrinoids which is a group of
cobalt-containing compounds that, in humans, are active
biologically.

In foods of animal origin such as shellfish, dairy
products, liver, meat and fish, you can mainly find

vitamin B_{12}. For vegans, plant-based milk substitutes such as oat milk, soy milk and rice milk are often enriched with vitamin B_{12}, and might therefore be an important product for vegans (129).

In foods, vitamin B_{12} is bound to a protein, and through the action of pepsin and hydrochloric acid in the stomach, the protein is cleaved from vitamin B_{12} and then vitamin B_{12} is re-bound to haptocorrin (transcobalamin I). Vitamin B_{12} cannot be absorbed without a glycoprotein that is secreted in the stomach's parietal cells and is called intrinsic factor. When vitamin B_{12} arrives to the small intestine, it binds to the intrinsic factor after it has released from haptocorrin, and this complex (vitamin B_{12} bound to intrinsic factor) is absorbed in the ileum by special receptors. In the enterocytes, vitamin B_{12} is bound to transcobalamin II, and now the complex can be called holotranscobalamin, it enters the blood circulation and is quickly taken up by bone marrow, liver and other tissues. In the circulation, most of the vitamin B_{12} is bound to transcobalamin I and can be stored for many days while holotranscobalamin only can be stored for about an hour.

At intakes between 1.5 micrograms to 2.0 micrograms per meal, the ileal receptors are saturated, but if the intake increases, it results in reduced percentage of absorbed vitamin B_{12}. Healthy adults with normal gastric function tend to absorb 50 % of dietary vitamin B_{12}. 2 – 5 milligrams of vitamin B_{12} is stored in the body and half of this amount is stored in the liver. Around 0.1 % of vitamin B_{12} is lost daily from the total body pool (130,131).

If you have stomach ulcer, your absorption will get worse. Some older people have lack of the intrinsic factor which makes it harder to absorb vitamin B_{12}.
When vitamin B_{12} has bounded with the intrinsic factor, it is transported to the blood where it is transported with the transport protein transcobalamin to the tissues where it interacts with folate. The bile allows vitamin B_{12} to be reabsorbed in the terminal ileum which means that the enterohepatic circulation must work well. The vitamin B_{12} can be stored in the body for 5 – 10 years (108).

Vitamin B_{12} is responsible for the amino acid metabolism, the conversion of homocysteine to methionine where tetrahydrofolate is needed, neurological functions, fatty acid metabolism and the interaction with the C1-group in the production of RNA and DNA with folate (108).

If you don't consume enough of vitamin B_{12}, it can lead to peripheral neuropathy, homocysteine anemia, neurological dysfunctions such as depression, cognition problems, multiple sclerosis and schizophrenia. Shortage can also lead to pernicious anemia which is terrible and means that the erythrocytes (red blood cells) are diminished, but this disease is seen very rarely (108). Deficiency symptoms only occur after several years of low intake of vitamin B_{12} or through decreased absorption, so the symptoms of vitamin B_{12} deficiency is rare for most people (130). Vitamin B_{12} deficiency symptoms often occur through vitamin B_{12} malabsorption, which often results from persons who have hypochlorhydria (lack of stomach acid) and atrophic gastritis (131).

The people that are in a higher risk of developing these symptoms and diseases are the people that are vegans and the elderly people because they often have gastric ulcer and lack of intrinsic factor and lack of hydrochloric acid which can lead to neuropathy which is incurable.

You can find vitamin B_{12} in fish, seafood, liver, meat, eggs, milk and cheese (108).

Recommendations of vitamin B_{12}

The recommended intake for both men and women is 2 micrograms per day. The lowest recommended intake for both men and women is 1 microgram per day and the highest recommended intake for both men and women is not established (129). Studies have proven that an intake of vitamin B_{12} over 100 micrograms per day from supplements and foods does not represent a health risk, and, therefore, there is no highest recommended intake of vitamin B_{12} (132).

The three next nutrients I will describe are so-called macronutrients, which include carbohydrates, protein and fat.

Carbohydrates

Carbohydrates give us energy, they are starting materials for nucleic acids, non-essential amino acids and glucuronic acid (detoxification, bile acid) but also amino sugar (glycoproteins glucoseaminoglucans) that is important for connective tissue cartilage, signaling and the immune system (133).

Now, I am going to describe different forms of carbohydrates, so just keep up with the reading.

The three major carbohydrate groups are sugars that consist of 1 or 2 monomers, oligosaccharides that consist of 3 to 9 monomers and polysaccharides that consist of 10 or more monomers. The most important sources of carbohydrates in foods are lactose, sucrose and trehalose (disaccharides), fructose, galactose and glucose (monosaccharides), polysaccharides (starch – the main forms are amylopectin and amylose and non-starch polysaccharides – the main forms are hemicelluloses, hydrocolloids, cellulose and pectins) and oligosaccharides (134).

We start with High Fructose Corn Syrup (HFCS) that is a hydrolysis of corn starch. HFCS is made from an isomerization of glucose to fructose (55 %).

Next one is glycose that is wheat starch which has partially been broken down to maltodextrins and glucose.

Next one is lactose (milk sugar). Some people are lactose intolerant which means that they have a reduced production of the enzyme lactase. Lactose intolerance is common in the world. Lactose intolerance may cause diarrhea, bloating, production of gas and osmotic effects in the stomach.

Maltose and sucrose are broken down in the body to fructose, glucose and 2 glucose in the intestinal mucosa membrane by enzymes. Maltose and sucrose are transported to the liver by the hepatic portal system. Glucagon and insulin (GLUT4) regulates the glucose level of the blood.

Starch is a mixture of two forms of glucose polymers (amylopectin and amylose). Starch is also the main carbohydrate storage form of the plants.

Glycogen is a branched glucose polymer that looks like amylopectin. Glycogen is the main carbohydrate storage form in animals. When the liver and muscles need to get rid of energy, the glycogen get activated very fast from the cytoplasm. The body digests amylopectin faster than amylose.

Vitargo is another form of glycogen that is a very large branched starch molecule which gives the body very much glucose but it won't affect the osmotic balance (133).

The glycemic carbohydrates which means "providing carbohydrate for metabolism" include sucrose and lactose (disaccharides), fructose and glucose (monosaccharides), starch (polysaccharide) and malto-oligosaccharides (134) (gives a blood glucose response) are broken down in the body by different enzymes. Amylase, found in the saliva breaks down starch. Amylase also found in pancreatic juice keeps up with the breakdown of starch. Maltase, lactase and saccharase, found in the intestinal juices break down disaccharides into monosaccharides which are transported to the bloodstream (133). Glucose and fructose are mainly found in berries, fruits, some vegetables and juices, and these carbohydrates provide sucrose which is mainly found in sweets and soft drinks. Lactose is mainly found in milk products and milk. Malto-oligosaccharides are mainly found in partially hydrolyzed starch. Starch is mainly found in tubers, potatoes, cereal products and bread (135).

Monosaccharides are transported through the hepatic portal system to the liver which fills up the glycogen storage. The glucose is transported to the blood circulation and the galactose is converted into glucose in the liver and fructose is converted into glucose or fat in the liver. The blood glucose level is around $4 - 5.5$ mmol / L.

Glucose or galactose and sodium ions (Na^+) are collected by SGLT1. Fructose is collected by GLUT5. When the galactose, glucose and fructose are in the cell, GLUT2 helps with the transportation into the bloodstream. All these processes cost ATP (energy) (133).

The characterization of fructose is that a high intake of fructose can cause increased levels of blood lipids and increased fat storage in the liver. When we consume more energy than the body expends, fructose is converted to fat in the liver when glucose is present. When fat is produced, it stimulates the formation of VLDL (133).

Another form of carbohydrates is polysaccharides which can be in the form of digestible and indigestible. The digestible polysaccharides are characterized in the way that they can be broken down by the gastrointestinal tract enzymes. The carbohydrates that can be broken down are glycogen and starch and it is only these that can raise the blood sugar. The indigestible polysaccharides are characterized in the way that they cannot be broken down by the gastrointestinal tract. The carbohydrates that cannot be broken down are dietary fiber, cellulose and resistant starch (133).

Another form of carbohydrates is dietary fiber which consists of resistant oligosaccharides (galacto-oligosaccharides, fructo-oligosaccharides and other resistant oligosaccharides), non-starch polysaccharides (hemicelluloses, hydrocolloids, pectin and cellulose), lignin and resistant starch (some types of raw starch granules, physically enclosed starch, chemically modified starches and retrograded amylose) (136).

If polyols are absorbed in excess amount in the small intestine, the results may be diarrhea. If fructose is consumed without glucose, it may also cause diarrhea (137).

Another form of carbohydrates is cellulose which consists of straight glucose chains, which produces dietary fibers that are held together by strong hydrogen bonds. Therefore, cellulose is not water-soluble (133).

Another form of carbohydrates is oligosaccharides that consist of beta-galactoside bonds which the human being cannot cleave which lead to gas formation in the microflora which lead to flatulence which lead to the production of SCFA (133).

Another form of carbohydrates is gel-forming dietary fibers. These have positively specific functions in the body. For example, the blood sugar increases slower, the stomach empties slower, the blood cholesterol level is reduced slightly, they bind bile salts and preventing them from returning to the liver, the liver removes blood cholesterol to produce more bile salts. You can find gel-forming dietary fibers in psyllium seeds, oatmeal, fruits and vegetables (133).

The blood glucose level is important for the body. The brain's main substrate is glucose which means that the brain cannot use fat or protein as energy sources. This means that the brain need an even flow of glucose (sugar). The blood sugar level is maintained even by hormones. Glucagon increases the release of glucose from the liver. Insulin increases the cells' uptake of glucose. Adrenaline increases the muscles' uptake of glucose. Incretins (GLP-1 and GIP) inhibit glucagon and stimulate insulin (133). The blood glucose level is determined by 1) how fast the carbohydrates are taken up in the body, 2) the elimination or the net liver uptake, and 3) glucose uptake in the peripheral (138).

When the blood glucose level is lowered (hypoglycemia), it causes reduced gluconeogenesis and increased production of glycogen in the liver. The body can handle low blood glucose levels through regeneration of glucose from lactic acid, degradation of liver glycogen to glucose, gluconeogenesis from glycerol and glucogenic amino acids in the liver and in the kidneys, and through glycerol from degradation which can only give ketone bodies which can be used by the brain when there is not enough of glucose (133).

When we read about carbohydrates, we can see something called Glycemic Index (GI) which is how fast different foods give an insulin response in the body. If the GI is high, it gives you a fast insulin response and if the GI is low, it gives you a slow insulin response. The reference intake that determines GI is 50 g of glucose.

The food's GI level is affected by the cellular structure (if it is whole grain which gives a low insulin response or if it is a white bread which gives a fast insulin response), amylopectin / amylose ratio, sugars, crystallization – retrogradation, organic acids, amylase inhibitors and viscosity (the gelatinization degree) (133).

When we talk about carbohydrates, we should name something about the intestinal flora (our intestinal bacteria). The intestinal flora has a weight of 1 – 1.5 kg (2.22 – 3.33 lbs). There are around 1000 different species where the most of them are in the large intestine. The bacteria live on substances that cannot be broken down and absorbed in the small intestine. The intestinal flora is of very importance for the overall health (133).

When we talk about carbohydrates, we should also cover what the fermentable dietary fibers produce. They produce SCFA (many have positive health effects), antimicrobials, gases, increased drainage volume, faster pass time and increased number of good bacteria.

While on the other hand, non-fermentable dietary fibers cause increased drainage volume, faster pass time and it binds water. Non-fermentable dietary fiber is in the form of cellulose and it stimulates peristalsis which reduces the risk of pocketing and constipation. It also gives bulk to the intestinal bacteria.

Dietary fibers also produce some fermentation products which are the SCFA propionate, acetic acid and butyrate which are absorbed in the colon. Propionate decreases the production of cholesterol, butyrate provides nutrition to the intestinal mucosa which gives us a good health in the bowel, acetic acid provides energy to tissues and muscles. Dietary fibers also cause lower pH which leads to less production of cancerogenic substances (133).

When we now are talking about dietary fibers, it is a perfect moment to tell you why it is unhealthy for you to consume too little dietary fibers. Too little consumption of dietary fibers can lead to development of diabetes, development of small intestine cancer, development of cardiovascular diseases, constipation and risk of overweight (133).

Something interesting about carbohydrates is that if you consume too much carbohydrates, it will inhibit the fat oxidation and fat degradation (fat burning process). This means that we shouldn't consume too much carbohydrates when we want to lose weight, but when we want to build muscles and get bigger, then carbohydrates are excellent to consume in a bigger amount. But one thing is for sure, you need carbohydrates in your diet so your body can function well.

A too low intake of carbohydrates can be beneficially sometimes. A low carbohydrate intake will lead to weight loss, but as I wrote earlier in the book, the weight reduction will almost be the same whether you consume more carbohydrates or if you consume less carbohydrates. In a lot of magazines, you can see a person that says, "I lost 6 kg (13.33 lbs) in just one week". Do you think that is true? I know it's true, because if you stop to consume carbohydrates, or consume very few carbohydrates, it will give you a fast weight loss because you will lose water that are bounded in glycogen. To consume too little carbohydrates during a long period of time is unhealthy for your body! When you lose weight, the blood sugar level and cholesterol levels are positively affected (133).

How does the body digest carbohydrates?

The long carbohydrate chains are cleaved into disaccharides by the enzyme alpha-amylase in saliva and pancreas. The digestion of the carbohydrates starts in the saliva and keeps on in the small intestine where the pancreas secretes pancreatic juice that contains a lot of alpha-amylase, and it is also here the largest part of the carbohydrates are digested. Enzymes in the microvilli in the small intestine help to break down disaccharides into monosaccharides in the form of galactose, glucose and fructose, and it is these monosaccharides that we absorb. All these three forms of monosaccharides will pass the microvilli's epithelial cells, but galactose and glucose will be absorbed by secondary active transport that is sodium dependent in the epithelial cells, while fructose will pass through to the epithelial cells by facilitated diffusion. Through facilitated diffusion, galactose, glucose and fructose leave the epithelial cells and are transported to the liver via the hepatic portal system. After the monosaccharides have been transported to the liver, they go out in the blood circulation through the blood vessel called vena cava inferior (32).

Recommended intake of carbohydrates

The recommended intake of carbohydrates is 45 – 60 % of the total energy intake. Added sugars should be kept below 10 % of the total energy intake and dietary fibers should be 25 grams / day or more for women and 35 grams / day or more for men, according to NNR 2012 (139).

The major sources of carbohydrates should be whole fruits, pulses, whole-grain cereals, vegetables, seeds and nuts. The recommended carbohydrate intake of 45 – 60 % of the total energy intake is the best range for reducing the risk of chronic diseases. A sufficient intake of dietary fibers help to reduce the risk of constipation and contributes to a decreased risk of type-2 diabetes, cardiovascular disease and colorectal cancer, it also helps to maintain a healthy body weight (140).

The intake of added refined sugars (fructose, sucrose, starch hydrolysates like high-fructose syrup and glucose syrup and other isolated sugar preparations used as manufacturing or food preparation) should be less than 10 % of the total energy intake due to ensure sufficient intake of dietary fibers and micronutrients which are very important for individuals who are losing body weight due to a low-calorie intake and for children. The intake of sugar-sweetened beverages increase the risk of dental caries, excess weight gain and type-2 diabetes and due to these evidences, the total intake of sugars should be limited to less than 10 % of the total energy intake (141).

Carbohydrates and glycemic carbohydrates related to body weight

Systematic reviews and meta-analysis have showed that an increased intake of sugar is associated with weight gain while a reduced intake of sugar is associated with weight reduction among adults.

Another systematic review and meta-analysis of 33 randomized controlled trials showed that a reduced fat intake (28 – 43 % of the total energy intake) resulted in less weight gain of 1.4 – 1.6 kg (3.11 lbs – 3.55 lbs). The NNR 2012 systematic review showed that the proportion of macronutrients had little influence on the treatment of obesity, while fewer meats, refined grains, sugar-rich foods and beverages and plenty of dairy products and fiber-rich foods were associated with a lower body weight.

Meta-analyses have shown that high-protein, low-carbohydrate diets resulted in lower body weight or similar body weight compared to diets reduced in fat up to six months. Long-term effects of low-carbohydrate diets related to body weight are less clear (142,143).

Dietary fiber-rich foods have effects such as slower gastric emptying, diminishes energy density, decreases rate of nutrient absorption and have short-term increase in satiety. These effects of the dietary fiber-rich foods might play an important role when it comes to body weight reduction (144). There are probable evidences that the body weight among adults are reduced when the intake of dietary fibers in the diet are increased (145).

The major sources of dietary fibers should come from whole fruits, pulses, wholegrain cereals, nuts and vegetables (146).

Protein

There are 20 + 1 common amino acids where the +1 is selenocysteine. The amino acids are grouped according to the side chains properties on the amino acids which can be polar, hydrophobic, modified (special case), positively charged and negatively charged.

Amino acids are also Zwitterions which means that they both have a positive charge and a negative charge and are also water soluble.

Proteins are built up by peptide bonds (chain of amino acids) which are created between an amino group and a carboxyl group, are created with the help of the cell's ribosomes and are relatively stable. Common peptide bonds are hydrolyzed by proteases such as trypsin, pepsin and carboxypeptidase while peptide bonds between side chains are not hydrolyzed by food digestive enzymes (147).

Proteins can have four different structures; primary structure, secondary structure, tertiary structure and quaternary structure. The primary structure is about the order of the amino acids and is determined by the gene of the protein (a DNA-code). The secondary structure is about regular repeating patterns in the structure which depends on hydrogen bonds. Two common structures in the secondary structure is alpha helix and beta structure. The tertiary structure is about how the entire peptide chain is folding which depends on the links between the side chains. The last structure, the quaternary structure, is about interactions and form between two or more subunits in a protein, for example, A2B2: 2 pieces of A subunits and 2 pieces of B subunits (147).

How does the degradation and uptake of protein work?

Proteins from food are broken down in the small intestine and in the stomach to free amino acids (largest part), di- and tripeptides and oligopeptides (by oligopeptidases). These broken-down proteins are absorbed mostly in the small intestine's mucosa cells. The peptides in the small intestine are taken up by PEPT1, peptides in the kidneys are taken up by PEPT2 and the peptides are transported with H^+.

The body takes up peptide and amino acid blend faster than just pure amino acid blend (147).

Different proteins have different nutritional values due to different amino acid content. If you don't consume enough of all the essential amino acids, it can lead to a negative nitrogen-balance. If you consume vegetable foods with amino acids, you may lack some of the essential amino acids because there is not enough of essential amino acids in vegetable foods. On the other hand, animal foods with amino acids contain sufficient essential amino acids for the body's needs (147).

Some amino acids are inaccessible such as amino acids that are not released by digestion. The biggest problem when it comes to amino acids are lysine because it is very restrictive in many nutrionally proteins, it has an E-amino group that can create a peptide bond with a carboxyl side chain which cannot be broken down by the enzymes in the stomach and the small intestine (147).

If you consume too much proteins, the excess amino acids are not stored, instead, they are broken down by either deamination (the amino group is removed and forms urea) or that the carbon skeleton is taken care of. The carbon skeleton can be disintegrated in two different ways, depending on the final product. The first way and final product is glucogenous amino acids which means that the skeletonl is metabolized to oxaloacetate or pyruvate which can be converted to glucose through the gluconeogenesis. The second way and final product is ketogenic amino acids which means that the skeleton is metabolized to acetoacetyl-CoA or acetyl-CoA which can be converted to ketone cells (147).

You can find proteins mostly in meat, dairy products and cereals (147).

The population reference intake for protein is for older adults 0.83 grams / kg of body weight per day and for infants, children and adolescents between 0.83 grams and 1.31 grams / kg of body weight per day depending on the age (147).

We always lose some of the proteins we consume daily, approximately 10 g protein / day of approximately 150 – 200 g protein / day are lost when we do our needs in the toilet. These lost 10 g of proteins can be through non-degraded proteins from the diet, mucosal cells, intestinal bacteria and mucus which is difficult to break down and is stable.

Around 16.5 % of the protein is nitrogen and nitrogen we lose from urine, feces, dead skin cells, hair and sweat. There can be a positive and a negative nitrogen balance. A positive nitrogen balance means that the intake of nitrogen is higher than the losses which leads to anabolism (the building phase) which is important for growing children. A negative nitrogen balance means that the intake is lower than the losses which leads to catabolism (the break down phase) which can be caused by a trauma, protein deficiency in the diet or by an infection.

The nitrogen balance is negative during fasting/starvation and is positive after a meal.

If you don't consume enough proteins it can lead to cachexia which is muscle atrophy and emaciation. The symptoms of cachexia are decreased production of protein and increased break down of protein. Cachexia may be seen in older people, HIV patients, cancer patients, people who have anorexia and of course when the protein intake is too low.

If you want to have a good nitrogen balance then you must increase your protein intake (147).

How does the body digest proteins?

The proteins begin to digest in the stomach where the most important protein-degrading enzyme is called pepsinogen which get activated by hydrochloric acid into pepsin (the active enzyme that digest proteins). No digestion of proteins take place in the saliva. Another important enzyme when it comes to proteins is pancreatic trypsinogen which get activated by enterocinases in the small intestine, and its function is to activate inactive zymogens that are released from the pancreas such as chymotrypsin and trypsin (digest proteins). 20 different aminopeptidases (found in the epithelial cells' luminal membranes) together with trypsin, pepsin and chymotrypsin digest proteins. There are now different long peptide chains in the lumen that we pick up with the help of secondary active transport linked to Na^+ which results in that the amino acids go to the epithelial cell. Only one amino acid can be cleaved at once and be taken up by the epithelial cell. The aminopeptidases help to cleave the peptides (if it is, for example, three of them, called tripeptide). Dipeptides and tripeptides can also be taken up and be digested in the epithelial cell and become free amino acids through a hydrolysis of the peptide bonds. The transport of this system is called secondary active transport that is connected to the H^+-gradient. Via facilitated diffusion, the amino acids are transported from the epithelial cells to the hepatic portal system, from the hepatic portal system, the amino acids are transported to the liver (32).

Recommended intake of protein

The recommended protein intake is 10 – 20 % of the total energy intake which corresponds to about 0.8 – 1.5 g protein / kg body weight per day for adults, according to NNR 2012 (148).

Protein related to body weight, muscle mass, strength and physical exercise

It has been proven that participants experience higher satiety after protein intake than after fat intake and carbohydrate intake. A systematic review which analyzed low-calorie/high-protein diets from year 1966 to 2003 related to weight loss, showed that only the low-calorie intake was associated with weight loss and not the protein intake.

The proportion of macronutrients in the diet does not affect changes in waist circumference or body weight. According to NNR 2012, there is insufficient data on protein intake in obese/overweight participants related to weight reduction for an establishment (149,150).

Most of the systematic reviews show that less lean body mass is lost when the protein intake is between 13 – 20 % of the total energy intake (149).

According to the position statement, athletes who performs endurance and strength training should consume a protein intake between 1.2 – 1.7 grams per kg body weight, but in healthy adults who perform regular physical activity, the protein intake does not have to be increased because there is little evidence on this area (151).

A short-term study proved that the muscle protein synthesis after an exercise increased as much of 30 grams of protein as 90 grams of protein in the meal after an exercise (152).

Fat

The first question I will ask and give you an answer to is: why do we need fat?

Fat protects internal organs, stores energy in the fatty tissue as energy reserves, build and repair cells, surfactant to reduce the lungs' tension, adiponectin and leptin are produced by the fatty tissue, starting material for steroid hormones such as estrogen, testosterone, progesterone and cortisol, aldosterone and dehydroepiandrosterone (DHEA) and fat is also important for the uptake of the fat-soluble vitamins A, D, E and K (153).

When you consume too much energy (calories), the excess calories will be stored in fat cells as triglycerides in normal weighted individuals. In obese individuals, the excess calories can also be stored in the liver, muscles and pancreas. The triglycerides are produced in the liver, enterocytes, fat cells and mammary glands during lactation by esterification of three fatty acids into a glycerol skeleton. A triglyceride is built up by three esterified fatty acids bounded to a glycerol. The three esterified fatty acids can be unsaturated, saturated, cis form, trans form and branched carbon chain (153).

The fat can also be in the form of phospholipids which can be in two forms, either phosphoglycerides which are built up by two fatty acids and an ester of glycerol or sphingolipids which are built up by a fatty acid and an ester of sphingosine (153).

The fat can also be in the form of cholesterol which is present esterified with a fatty acid or in free form. But why is cholesterol important to us? Cholesterol stabilizes cell membrane, it is starting material for bile acids and steroid hormones, it is produced in the liver by the enzyme HMG-CoA reductase, but it can also be produced in all cells that have a nucleus, it is absorbed from the intestine and incorporated into the chylomicrons in the enterocytes, it is absorbed with the help of NPC1L1 in the intestine and the excess cholesterol is lost through feces (153).

The cholesterol's degradation happens in the way that cholesterol is oxidized by the liver to different bile salts through conjugation to taurine, glycine, sulphate or glucuronic acid. 5 % of the cholesterol is lost through feces and 95 % of the cholesterol returns to the enterohepatic cycle. The cholesterol can be transported to the liver in either one of two ways, the first way is that

HDL transports cholesterol directly to the liver and the second way is that HDL leaves the cholesterol to IDL or chylomicrons which take cholesterol to the liver (153).

When we consume foods with fat, enzyme-rich pancreas and bile that contains cholesterol, 95 % water and xenobiotics are secreted. The bile emulsifies the fat, the bile salts activate cholesterol esterase and when the concentration of the bile is high, a micell will be created (outer part of phospholipids, internal hydrophobic part with monoglycerides, cholesterol and free fatty acids) (153).

When the fat needs to be digested, some enzymes are needed for this process. The first enzyme is lipase that comes from gastric juice and saliva which hydrolyses triglycerides to free fatty acids, monoglycerides and glycerol. The second enzyme is phospholipases that hydrolyze phospholipids. The third and last enzyme is cholesterol esterase that hydrolyses cholesterol esters which lead to the creation of a fatty acid, free cholesterol, triglycerides, phospholipids and esters of fat-soluble vitamins (153).

The fat is absorbed in the upper part of the small intestine which is pleated with microvilli and villi for surface enlargement. In the villi, there is lymph nodes and blood vessels. Short-chain fatty acids are transported with albumin in the hepatic portal system because they have been hydrolyzed by the intestinal cell lipase. Lipids in the form of monoglycerides, free fatty acids and cholesterol are transported to the enterocytes via carrier-mediated transport or passive diffusion after they have passed the membrane. Only monoglycerides and free fatty acids pass the membrane to 100 % while cholesterol only passes the membrane to 50 %.

On the other hand, long chain fatty acids are re-esterified with glycerol and together with apolipoproteins, phospholipids and cholesterol, they are all packed together into something called chylomicrons which are large vesicles that are transported to the lymph for further transportation to the blood. Chylomicrons contain B-48 and E (34, 100). In the blood circulation, ApoC2 (connects lipoprotein lipase with the chylomicrons) is connected to the chylomicrons. A hydrolysis, that starts after two to three minutes after the chylomicrons have been transported to the blood circulation, around 50 % of the triglycerides from the chylomicrons have been released, where triglycerides release free fatty acids during the transportation in the blood is needed for chylomicrons to get into cells. The triglycerides can either be used by muscles during a muscle contraction or are stored in fat cells (153).

The fat is transported in the blood via different lipoproteins which are built up by phospholipids, cholesterol, proteins, a water-soluble surface, a fat-soluble inner core of cholesterol esters, triglycerides, esters of fat-soluble vitamins and apolipoproteins. All the chylomicrons are transported to muscles as energy substrates or to fatty tissues for storage (153).

There are some important hormones that control the fat metabolism, these hormones are glucagon, growth hormone, adrenaline, cortisol and insulin. Glucagon stimulates ketogenesis, growth hormone stimulates lipolysis, adrenaline stimulates lipolysis, cortisol stimulates lipolysis and insulin inhibits lipolysis.

There is also a hormone called hormone sensitive lipase (HSL) that is inhibited by insulin and activated by adrenaline and catalysts degradation of triglycerides to free fatty acid glycerol. Another important hormone is lipoprotein lipase (LPL) that hydrolyses triglycerides to free fatty acids and monoglycerides.

Another important hormone is Low Density Lipoprotein (LDL) that is responsible for the production of cholesterol in the cells and the transportation of cholesterol to the cells. LDL is built up by 45 % of cholesterol. Apo-B100 binds to receptors of LDL and is produced in the liver.

High Density Lipoprotein (HDL) is another important hormone when it comes to fat, and HDL is a small particle that is built up by 24 % phospholipids, 50 % protein, 22 % cholesterol and ApoA1. HDL transports triglycerides and excess cholesterol in the blood and tissues to the liver.

Very Low Density Lipoprotein (VLDL) is another important hormone that is built up by Apo-B100, E (34,100) and C-II by HDL when it comes to the blood circulation. VLDL distributes lipids for immediate use or storage and is produced in the liver of what is available. The content of VLDL depends on the contents in HDL, LDL, rest of chylomicrons, lipogenesis in the liver and fatty acids transported by albumin. LPL hydrolyzes triglycerides in VLDL and passes gradually to IDL before 50 – 60 % of IDL transforms to LDL. The rest, 40 – 50 % of IDL is absorbed in the liver. If you consume a lot of carbohydrates, the production of VLDL increases. There is also NPC1L1, that is very important when it comes to fat. NPC1L1 is needed for the uptake of cholesterol, is upregulated when we consume small amounts of cholesterol and is important for the uptake of plant sterols and cholesterol.

CD36, which is a receptor, is also important when it comes to fat. CD36 is more expressed when we consume a diet rich on fat, it is also more expressed in the fatty tissue in people that have diabetes type II. CD36 is important for taking up free fatty acids for energy use in the muscles and for storage in fatty tissues. CD36 can be found on transverse muscles and fatty tissues (153).

Fat can come into the body through two pathways, the first one is the endogenous lipoprotein pathway and the second one is the exogenous lipoprotein pathway. The endogenous lipoprotein pathway means that fat, as lipoproteins, are stored in the liver so it can be transported to the blood circulation or are produced in the liver. The exogenous lipoprotein pathway, on the other hand, means that the fat comes into the blood through the food and under influence of LPL, the chylomicrons are converted into rests of chylomicrons that are absorbed in the liver. In the intestinal tract's epithelial cells, chylomicrons are produced (153).

The production of chylomicrons is changed in different conditions of illness. For example, a high production of lipoprotein particles and / or a dysfunction of LPL can cause postprandial lipidemia, which can be seen in people with diabetes type 2, obesity, cardiovascular diseases and insulin resistance.

If you have a high number of triglycerides in the blood and many rests of chylomicrons in the blood, you can have an increased risk of cardiovascular diseases. High levels of triglycerides in the postprandial section, can be a higher risk of cardiovascular disease, but not when a person is fasting! The amount of triglycerides is controlled by two factors, the amount of chylomicrons (contribute the most) and the amount of VLDL.

The rests of the chylomicrons can even cause atherosclerosis by penetrating the vessel wall (153).

We have a fat metabolism in the liver. The liver is responsible for the production of VLDL, cholesterol and HDL. It is also the center of the lipid metabolism. The liver takes up rests of chylomicrons and LDL and can also store, form and export triglycerides. The liver is also responsible for the production of ketone bodies through fatty acid oxidation that connects the citric acid cycle with the fat metabolism (153).

Something very interesting about fat is that normal weighted individuals have more receptors for fat which causes these individuals to feel saturation earlier than individuals that are obese or overweight because those individuals have fewer receptors for fat. This can be a reason why people with obesity can eat a lot of food, especially high fat food, they have fewer receptors for fat. When you lose weight, the receptors for fat will be fewer and you will start to feel more saturated earlier when you consume fatty foods (153).

How does the body digest fat?
To make fat drops become smaller, we need to make sure the fat drops are mixed with bile salts. To get bile salts, we need to release bile (phospholipids are also released at the same time) to the fat in the food and to the small intestine. When this happens, the fat drops will be emulsified due to increased surface of the fat. What makes the food (cymus) mixed together are the bowel movements, phospholipids and bile salts. An enzyme called lipase which comes from the pancreas digests fat into free fatty acids and monoglycerides (a fatty acid bounded to a glycerol skeleton) which both produces micelles. The micelles do something called micelle

formation, it is when the micelles turn their fatty acids into each other. It is only the free fatty acids and monoglycerides that can be absorbed by the fat which transports easily through diffusion to the monoglycerides and free fatty acids. So, the lipase, helps to release the free fatty acids and monoglycerides from the fat drop which consists of triglycerides (three fatty acids bounded to a glycerol skeleton). The lipase cleaves two of three fatty acids on the glycerol skeleton, which leaves us with one fatty acid, called a monoglyceride, which is absorbed to the intestine's epithelial cells. When the free fatty acids and monoglycerides diffuse into the epithelial cell (enterocytes), they will be resynthesized into triglycerides again with the help of enzymes in the endoplasmic reticle of the cell. The triglycerides will be packed into a small membrane vesicle (chylomicrons) that is transported through exocytosis to the lacteal in the villus and further, diffuses into the lymph nodes in a blind lymphatic system which is transported, collected and emptied in the key bone vein. Notice here, that the fat is not being transported to the hepatic portal system, instead it ends up in the lymphoma and keeps on being transported directly to the bloodstream. It is only the SCFAs that can be directly transported to the liver, but not the long-chain fatty acids (32).

There is gastric lipase in the stomach, lingual lipase in the mouth and pancreatic lipase in the pancreas where all are important for fat absorption and fat digestion, but the pancreatic lipase is the most important. When we consume fat, we stimulate the production of CCK that releases bile and enzymes from the pancreas via a sphincter called Oddi's sphincter. The triglycerides in the chylomicrons will be digested to free fatty acids by enzymes, and these free fatty acids can be used to store excess fat in fat tissues or use it in muscle work. The chylomicrons end up in the lymph fluid (lacteals) (32).

Recommended intake of fat and fatty acids

The recommended intake of total fat is 25 – 40 % of the total energy intake, according to the NNR 2012. The recommended intake of monounsaturated fat is 10 – 20 % of the total energy intake, polyunsaturated fat is recommended to be 5 – 10 % of the total energy intake, n-3 (omega-3) fat should be kept equal to or over 1 % of the total energy intake, saturated fatty acids should be kept below 10 % of the total energy intake and trans-fatty acids should be as low as possible, according to NNR 2012 (154).

The NNR 2012 recommends that the saturated fatty acids should be replaced with monounsaturated fatty acids (oleic acid) and polyunsaturated fatty acids from vegetable dietary sources such as rapeseed oils or olive for reducing the concentrations of serum LDL-cholesterol. Reduction of the LDL/HDL-cholesterol ratio and the risk of coronary heart disease is seen when trans-fatty acids or saturated fatty acids are replaced with monounsaturated fatty acids and polyunsaturated fatty acids (155).

The NNR 2012 does not recommend that the total fat intake should be reduced below 25 % of the total energy intake due to the increasing concentrations of triglycerides in serum and the risk of impaired glucose tolerance and the risk of reducing HDL-cholesterol but even for the difficulty to ensure sufficient intake of essential fatty acids and fat-soluble vitamins (156).

Fat and fatty acids related to body weight

According to intervention studies, the weight reduction on average is 1.4 – 1.6 kg (3.11 lbs – 3.55 lbs) from six months to eight years when participants consumed reduced fat-diets ad libitum. There is no evidence that the body weight is affected by the quality of fat (157).

Chapter 13

Calories, physical activity and weight loss

When it comes to losing weight, one important factor to remember is that losing one pound (0.45 kg) of fat takes about 3500 calories. So, if you want to lose 1 to 2 pounds (0.45 kg to 0.90 kg) a week, you must reduce the calorie intake with around 500 – 1000 calories under your maintenance level. But how do you know your maintenance level? It is easy to understand, you must write down all the food (solid food and liquids) you eat and drink in a day. To know how many calories there are in a product you can use the app called "MyFitnessPal" and scan the product and type in the amount of the product you consumed or you can just read the nutrition label and see how many calories the product contains per serving or per 100 grams. You must also know how many calories you burn when you are physical active. "MyFitnessPal", also have this function where you type in for how long time you exercised and what type of training you did. You can also buy a clock called "Fitbit" that tracks your heart rate during a day, it tracks the time you sleep, and much more. SuperTracker is also an alternative (158).

The recommended physical activity levels are 150 minutes (2 hours and 30 minutes) of aerobic activities like powerwalking with moderate intensity weekly combined with 2 days per week of muscle strengthening activities where you work the major muscle groups (breasts, hips, legs, abdomen, back, arms and shoulders). The more you are physical active the greater the health benefits are. Teens and children need at least 60 minutes of physical activity each day and it is very important that you as a parent encourage them to be active, you can be active with them, like go for a walk, take a ride on the bike, climb mountains, go for a shop, just do something to increase the level of physical activity each day.

Every person needs different amounts of calories because every person's body is unique. Therefore, if a doctor tells you that you need to consume 1800 calories a day to lose weight and you weight 250 pounds (112.5 kg) then you can't tell your friend who weights 133.33 lbs (60 kg) to also consume 1800 calories to lose weight.

You don't have to track calories years in and years out, you can just start your weight loss program by tracking calories and reading nutrition labels for the first two to three weeks and then you will better understand how many calories the food you usually consume contains (158). Me, for example, track calories every day because I find it funny and interesting except for when I go out for a dinner at a restaurant then it becomes way harder to know how many calories the food you consume contains.

A good question to cover in this chapter is if you consume food late in the evening or even in the night, will the calories from the food you consumed turn automatically into body fat? The answer on this question is, no! When you consume your calories during a day doesn't affect the body weight, the only thing that affects your body weight is the total amounts of calories you consume and the total calories you burn during physical activity in a day (24 hours) (158).

Another important thing to remember is that even if you are physically active, you can't consume as much calories as you want, because if, for example, your maintenance level is 2500 calories and you are physically active during a day and burn for example 450 calories, then you can't consume more calories than 2950 or else you will gain weight (158).

And the last thing during this chapter to mention is that also the behavior, genetic factors and environment can contribute to overweight and obesity (158).

Chapter 14

Good food selections based on NNR 2012

Vegetables and root vegetables

The first food selection I am going to write about is vegetables and root vegetables.

In this group, you find beans, green leafy vegetables, onions, peas, root vegetables, cabbage plants, potatoes and corn which all are either preserved vegetables, frozen and fresh. Cabbage plants and green leafy vegetables contain high concentrations of many minerals and vitamins, but the most root vegetables and vegetables contain folate, vitamin C, vitamin K, beta carotene (a form of vitamin A), fibers and potassium. They are also nutritious and have low energy content (159).

Legumes

In this group, you find legumes that are dried, frozen, fresh and preserved like chickpeas, black beans, white beans, black eye beans, kidney beans, yellow and green peas and green beans. Legumes contain starch, protein, fiber, low fat content, zinc, potassium, iron, magnesium, all the B-vitamins except vitamin B_{12} and folate (159).

Fruits and berries

In this group, you find frozen and fresh berries and fruits. Fruits and berries contain fiber, vitamin C, sucrose and monosaccharides (glucose and fructose) (159).

Nuts and seeds

In this group, you find walnuts, almonds, peanuts, pistachios, pine nuts, hazelnuts, cashew nuts, sunflower seeds and sesame seeds. Nuts and seeds contain magnesium, copper, vitamin E, niacin, vitamin B_6, zinc, potassium, protein, polyunsaturated- and monounsaturated fatty acids, antioxidants and fiber (159).

Health effects of vegetables, root vegetables, legumes, fruits and berries and nuts and seeds

All these food sources contain protein, and it has been shown that protein from vegetable foods can reduce the risk of mortality in hypertension and cardiovascular diseases. It has also been shown that 25 – 30 grams of soy protein per day can reduce the blood's levels of LDL-cholesterol.

The fat from vegetables contain mostly monounsaturated- and polyunsaturated fats which give more positive health effects than saturated fats.

All these food sources contain dietary fiber which pass to the large intestine where they are broken down by microorganisms in the intestinal flora to gases and short chain fatty acids. Some dietary fibers are broken down almost completely and these contribute to the growth of the intestinal flora. Other dietary fibers are less broken down and they bind water which increases the volume of the feces. There is a high content of amylose in legumes which leads to a slower uptake of glucose due to slow digestion in the intestine. The monosaccharides in fruits and berries result in a quickly use of these as a carbohydrate source.

These food sources contain, as said before, folate, and folate is very important for the human being. Folate is important for the production of RNA and DNA, the turnover of some amino acids and cell division. Deficiency of folate leads to a disrupted metabolism of protein, affects the cell division and results in blood loss. Fruits, berries and vegetables also contain bioactive substances like lycopene, polyphenols, phytoestrogens and lectins and antioxidants which protect against harmful oxidative stress.

Diets that contain big amounts of vegetables like legumes, root vegetables, vegetables and fruits lead to reduced risk of chronic diseases. These food sources also contribute to weight stability (159).

Cereals

In this group, you find pasta, bread, rice and grains. Cereals contain protein, carbohydrates and fiber. Flakes, bread and porridge contain thiamine, iron, niacin, riboflavin, vitamin B_6 and folate. Bread contain iron, folate, zinc and magnesium. The only source of whole grain is found in cereals (159).

Health effects of cereal products

Whole grain products are very important because they contain zinc, iron, magnesium, phosphorus, fibers, niacin, vitamin E, riboflavin, thiamine, vitamin B_6, bioactive substances and antioxidants. Cereal products are an important source of iron and iron exists in myoglobin that in the muscles and enzymes transport oxygen, and it also exists in hemoglobin that in the blood transports oxygen. When the synthesis of hemoglobin is reduced, which occurs when the body's stores of iron are empty, then iron malignancy occurs which can cause impairment and fatigue.

The uptake of zinc and iron can be affected by the content of phytic acid in whole grains. By fermentation, germination and soaking of whole grain, the phytic acid is partially broken down. Whole grain products contain more nutrients than refined cereals products.

Whole grain products are associated with protection against chronic diseases. A lower consumption of sifted flour as cereal products are associated with a healthy dietary pattern, because sifted flour might increase the risk of weight gain. On the other hand, whole grain products are indicated to protect against obesity and weight gain.

In a literature review, it was showed that breast cancer, colorectal cancer, type II diabetes and cardiovascular disease is reduced by a higher intake of dietary fiber. World Cancer Research Fund convinced that development of colorectal cancer is reduced by vegetable fibers. What should be noticed is that fiber-rich foods are not only whole grain products, but legumes and vegetables are too. An intake of low glycemic index foods may be important for individuals with a BMI over 25 and 30. It is truly an association between reduced risk of colorectal cancer, cardiovascular disease and type II diabetes with an intake of whole grain (159).

Food fat

In this group, you find oil used on sandwiches, in baking and in cooking. Spreadable fats contain monounsaturated fat, saturated fat and polyunsaturated fat. Butterfat contain vitamin A, vitamin D and vitamin E (159).

Health effects of food fat

Cold-pressed oils, hot-pressed oils and all vegetable oils contain tocopherol which is an antioxidant that protects against degradation of polyunsaturated fatty acids in the tissues.

From protein and carbohydrates, monounsaturated- and saturated fatty acids can be synthesized in the body, except alpha linolenic acid (n-3 "omega 3") and linoleic acid (n-6 "omega 6"). The skin's permeability of water is regulated by n-6. The nervous system's function is partially controlled by n-3 and n-6. In cell membranes, n-6 and n-3 are important components and from n-6 and n-3, other fatty acids with more double bonds and longer carbon chain can be created. A too high intake of polyunsaturated fatty acids can lead to impairment of immune function, increased oxidation in cells and increased bleeding tendency, therefore, the recommended intake of polyunsaturated fatty acids should be kept between 5 – 10 % of the total energy intake.

The risk of cardiovascular disease may be reduced if some of the saturated fatty acids are replaced with the same proportion of polyunsaturated fatty acids and monounsaturated fatty acids. Oilseed grease and coconut grease contain a lot of saturated fatty acids which should be replaced with fats from rapeseed oil and olive oil which contain many monounsaturated fatty acids without many saturated fatty acids.

When the proportion of saturated fatty acids decrease, and monounsaturated- and polyunsaturated fatty acids increase in the same proportion as the reduction of saturated fatty acids, LDL cholesterol and total cholesterol in plasma or serum decrease. The risk of cardiovascular disease also decreases when saturated fatty acids are replaced with monounsaturated- and polyunsaturated fatty acids because the rate of HDL/LDL cholesterol and LDL cholesterol are good markers for the risk of cardiovascular disease. The risk of atherosclerosis also increases of a higher concentration of LDL cholesterol in serum. Consuming more polyunsaturated- and monounsaturated fatty acids combined with less carbohydrates have not been proven to improve blood fats.

The evidences show that the risk of cardiovascular disease increases by trans fatty acids, and trans fatty acids can be found in mixtures of food fat that contain much of butter and in butter itself, but the levels of trans fatty acids are low (159).

Milk and milk products

In this group, you find sour milk, milk, yogurt, cream, cheese, crème fraiche and similar products. Sour milk, milk and yogurt contain vitamin A, saturated fat, calcium, vitamin D, riboflavin, vitamin B_{12}, potassium, phosphorus, zinc and selenium. Cheese, itself, contains saturated fat and calcium and less amounts of other minerals and vitamins. Milk and milk products also contain iodine (159).

Health effects of milk and milk products

Milk products like fish, eggs, meat and poultry contain full protein with essential amino acids that need to come from the food. Proteins are important for tissue repair, muscle work, immune systems, enzymatic activity and transportation of substances in the body.

In people over 65 years old, greater muscle mass have been observed when the protein intake was between 13 – 20 % of the total energy intake. It is also possibly, but not accepted yet, that the risk of total mortality increases when the protein intake increases from animal food. The risk of cardiovascular disease might increase when the intake of more fatty milk products increase because these products contain a high proportion of saturated fatty acids, and this means that these products will lead to a larger intake of saturated fatty acids and less intake of polyunsaturated fatty acids. On the other hand, lean milk products contain many minerals and vitamins and contain a limited proportion of saturated fatty acids. The risk of cardiovascular disease can also increase from trans fatty acids in animal products like butter, fat milk products and meat from ruminants, but also in some pastries and sweets from some countries in the world.

In milk and milk products, there are a high concentration of calcium, and the most important food source of calcium is from these products. Calcium is important when teeth and skeleton are formed, but also for nerve function and in blood coagulation. Calcium deficiency can lead to osteoporosis and growth inhibition.

Lean milk products are associated with a lower risk of chronic disease. There are also some weak evidences that the risk of hypertension, metabolic syndrome and stroke reduces of milk products. Lower risk of type II diabetes and lower risk of colorectal cancer might be associated with milk products. Some evidences show that lower weight gain is associated with increased intake of fat milk products, and this effect might be caused by the bioactive substances, protein and calcium in milk products. Other studies, do not show any association between lower weight gain and milk products, these studies only showed that there is lower weight gain if the individual is in caloric deficit.

The risk of cardiovascular disease can be decreased by a higher intake of unsaturated- and polyunsaturated fatty acids and a lower intake of saturated fatty acids, therefore, NNR 2012 recommends that fat milk products should be replaced with lean milk products (159).

Egg

In this group, you find eggs from birds and hens. Eggs contain small amounts of many minerals and vitamins like iron, vitamin B_6, vitamin A, vitamin D, potassium, selenium, calcium and magnesium (159).

Health effects of eggs

Eggs contain about 10 grams of fat per 100 grams and they also contain all the essential amino acids. The egg yolk contain iron, iodine, selenium, zinc, calcium, vitamin B_{12}, folate, riboflavin, vitamin D, vitamin A, vitamin E, polyunsaturated fatty acids and around 200 milligrams of cholesterol. Lower intakes of fat milk

products and meat will lead to an enough reduction of
cholesterol (159).

Fish and seafood

In this group, you find seafood, fish, caviar and rum. The
definition of lean fish, is fishes that contain below 2
grams of fat per 100 grams and the definition of fat fish,
is fishes that contain over 8 grams of fat per 100 grams.
Seafood contains food like scallops, blue mussels,
shrimps, crayfish, lobster and crab. Fish and seafood
contain vitamin B_{12}, vitamin D, protein, selenium, niacin,
polyunsaturated fatty acids and iodine (159).

Health effects of fish and seafood

Mackerel, herring and salmon contain EPA
(eicosapentaenoic acid) and DHA (docosahexaenoic acid)
which are n-3 fatty acids. Leaner fishes like lean cod fish
contain less fat, but contain more EPA and DHA than
mackerel, herring and salmon. The risk of cardiovascular
disease is possible to be reduced by long chain n-3 fatty
acids like EPA and DHA. Fish and seafood are important

food sources of vitamin D. If there is deficiency of vitamin D during a long period of time, it can lead to osteomalacia (bone softening) in adults and rackits (English disease) or cramps in children. Fish and eggs are also important food sources of iodine. Deficiency of iodine causes goiter, and if deficiency of iodine occurs during the fetal stage it can lead to impaired development of the physical development, nervous system and can results in mental development disturbance. Fish is also an important source to selenium, and selenium interacts with vitamin E, protects cells against oxidation and participates in immunological defense mechanisms. Deficiency of selenium can cause increased risk of cancer and changes of the heart muscle.

Fish is also an important source to vitamin B_{12}, and vitamin B_{12} exists only in animal foods. Vitamin B_{12} has important functions in the nervous system and in the cells' metabolism. Pernicious anemia and neurological symptoms are some symptoms of serious deficiency of vitamin B_{12}. Older people have lower absorption of vitamin B_{12}, and therefore, they have higher risk of developing deficiency of vitamin B_{12}.

The nutrients in fish have been suggested to have protective effects on type II diabetes, cardiovascular disease and cognitive function (159).

Bird, red meat and processed meat products

In this group, you find goose, turkey, chicken and other birds during the category bird. During the category red meat, you find lamb, pig, horse, beef and wild animals. During the category processed meat products, you find meat preserved by additives of chemical preservatives or by smoking, salt/nitrite. Red meat and meat dishes contain iron, zinc, several B-vitamins, selenium, vitamin D and protein. Chicken and chicken dishes contain niacin (159).

Health effects of bird, red meat and processed meat products

Red meat and birds contain, like said before, B-vitamins, zinc and iron, and are therefore nutritionally-friendly foods. Blood pudding, red meat and liver contain much iron, in the form of heme iron, which the body absorbs easier than non-heme iron which is found in vegetables. Unfortunately, a higher intake of heme iron is considered probable associated with a higher risk of chronic disease and type II diabetes.

A small proportion from meat like pigs, beefs, sheep and processed meat products from different kinds of meat is associated with lower risk of chronic disease.

Processed meat products and meat are associated with a higher risk of type II diabetes, according to population studies (159).

High concentrations of salt are often found in processed meat products, and cardiovascular disease and high blood pressure is associated with a high intake of salt. Increased risk of cardiovascular disease is associated with an intake of fatty processed meat products which contain much saturated fats. Increased risk of colorectal cancer is associated with a high intake of processed meat products and red meat. The risk of cancer increases when 500 grams of red meat and less grams of processed meat products are consumed per week. There is probably an association between weight gain and a high consumption of meat.

There are no evidences that the risk of colorectal cancer increases by intake of birds (159).

Salt and salty foods

In this group, you find salt (sodium chloride) used for optimizing the process for example baking, texture sensors and for preserving. Increase the flavor in foods is the biggest reason why salt is used in foods. You can find salt in processed meat products, salty snacks, herring deposits, but also in products like ready meals, cheese and bread (159).

Health effects of salt

The sodium ion is important for the regulation of the osmotic pressure in tissue fluid, blood plasma and for blood volume. Sodium is also important for the absorption of certain amino acids and glucose and for the normal functioning of the nerves. Deficiency of sodium is rare because there is sodium in many foods.

The risk of increased systolic- and diastolic blood pressure caused by salt intake is well associated. Hypertension can lead to cardiovascular disease. When individuals are reducing foods with salt, the blood pressure can be decreased. Adverse effects on renal functioning can be caused by a high intake of salt. Many salts have added iodine which is important for the health (159).

Energy-rich and sugar-sourced foods

In this group, you find foods that contain much added sugar but little fiber or much fat. They don't contain much minerals and vitamins, but they contain many calories. The products can be chocolate, candy, marmalade, jam, pastries and ice cream. The products can even be energy-rich drinks like juices, sports and energy drinks, soft drinks and sweet soups. Energy density means that the energy is given in relation to the weight in kJ per gram. For example, there is 20 kJ per gram in a chocolate cake, but it contains very few nutrients. Rapeseed oil contain 40 kJ per gram and contain also many important nutrients. Rapeseed oil is not included in this group, because it contributes to many minerals and vitamins (159).

Health effects of energy-rich and sugar-sourced foods

A high-energy intake of energy-rich- and sugar-sourced foods will lead to lower quality of the food due to lower density of the food. Over 10 % of added sugar of the total energy intake will lead to that the nutrients are more difficult to cover.

When the pH decreases due to breakdown of carbohydrates in the mouth by bacteria, caries occurs. The development of caries can be increased by sugar and starchy foods which contain carbohydrates that are easily degradable. Fluoride, meal composition and meal patterns can be important for the development of caries. A limitation of snacks that contain sugar and a limitation of refined sugar can decrease the risk of caries.

In a systematic literature review in NNR 2012, it was showed that the risk of diabetes type II probably increases of consumption of 2 bottles of soft drinks per week or two glasses of soft drinks per week or 2 jars of soft drinks per week. Consumption of soft drinks in these amounts probably lead to weight gain, because of the high-energy intake. Negative effects on blood fats and higher blood pressure is associated with consumption of soft drinks. There is an association between consumption of sweet desserts and candy and the risk of weight gain. Ice cream and pastries often contain a lot of saturated fatty acids and trans fatty acids and a high intake of saturated fatty acids and trans fatty acids can increase the risk of cardiovascular disease and therefore, it is better to replace saturated fatty acids and trans fatty acids with monounsaturated- and polyunsaturated fatty acids from vegetables.

Added sugar in the diet contribute to no health benefits (159).

Alcoholic beverages

In this group, you find alcoholic drinks like wine, folk beer, strong beer, spirits, soft drink, light beer and cider (159).

Health effects of alcoholic beverages

According to NNR 2012, women should not consume more than 10 grams of alcohol per day and men should not consume more than 20 grams of alcohol per day. The alcohol intake should not be over 5 % of the total energy intake. Alcohol reduces the foods' quality because there is not many minerals and vitamins in alcohol, and it also contains a lot of energy and some drinks also contain sugar.

Low and moderate intake of alcohol for middle- and older years old individuals decreases the risk of total mortality, but a high intake of alcohol increase the risk of total mortality in all age groups. When alcohol is consumed in a large amount during a short period of time, the risk of mortality increases in every individual. The risk of high blood pressure and cardiovascular disease probably increase of high intakes of alcohol. Ethanol is a carcinogen and the risk of many types of cancer increases of alcohol. In moderate intake of alcohol, the risk of breast cancer increases in women. Consumption of 70 grams per day of alcohol will cause alcohol damage. Individuals who consume high intakes of alcoholic beverages often have deficiency of thiamine, phosphorus, vitamin C, magnesium, protein and vitamin D (159).

Health effects of water

Water is important for the regulation of body temperature and for functions of many organs. The need for fluid is controlled by physical activity, individual factors and climate. At least 1 L of water in addition to the water from the food is needed for individuals (159).

The risk of increased blood clots and more viscous blood are dangerous effects of dehydration in combination with increased free fatty acid levels in the blood. When you are hydrated, the fat cells are effective when it comes to releasing fat, but when we are dehydrated, the fat cells are less effective in releasing fat. Increased muscle breakdown is an effect of dehydration; therefore, we should drink enough water when we are exercising and when we are in rest. Another result of dehydration is decreased insulin sensitivity which results in higher levels of insulin which leads to inhibition of fat burning. Decreased insulin sensitivity is a good factor for the development of diabetes type II. It is important to drink enough of water, around 2 L per day, but not in a short period of time (160).

Chapter 15

Research on food

Green tea

The plant of tea, *Camellia sinensis*, is grown in 30 countries. *Camellia sinensis* grows best in subtropical and tropical areas. In the world, it is produced, four types of tea from the same plant depending on the process of the tea leaves. The teas are green, white, black and oolong tea. The production of green tea comes from mature leaves that has been minimal processed (drying only). The production of white tea comes from buds and very young leaves that haven't turned green yet. The production of black tea comes from ripe leaves that are fully fermented. The production of oolong tea comes from ripe leaves that are partially fermented.

In Korea, China and Japan the consumption of green tea is most common. The production of green tea worldwide is about 20 % of the production of all teas. In Taiwan and China, the consumption of oolong tea is most common. In UK and US, the consumption of black tea is most common. The production of black tea worldwide is about 78 % of the production of all teas. The content of caffeine in black tea is up to three times as much as in green tea (161).

Medically seen, catechins which make up 80 – 90 % of the flavonoids, a type of polyphenols, are the most important component in green tea. In green tea, the catechins also make up around 40 % of the water-soluble solids. The amount of catechins in tea can be affected by where the leaves are grown, the growing conditions, how the leaves are processed, which leaves are harvested and how the tea is prepared. A disadvantage when tea is harvested is that the polyphenols are rapidly oxidized due to an enzyme called polyphenol oxidase, but to minimize the loss of polyphenols it is important to heat the leaves quickly by pan frying or steam to disable the enzyme polyphenol oxidase. The leaves in green tea are heated very quickly after harvest while the leaves in black tea are first dried, then rolled and crushed which promote oxidation. This means that green tea contains more catechins than black tea. In green tea, there are four main catechins which are Epigallocatechin-3-gallate (EGCG) which corresponds to approximately 59 % of total catechins, Epigallocatechin (EGC) which corresponds to approximately 19 % of total catechins, Epicatechin-3-gallate (ECG) which corresponds to approximately 14 % of total catechins and lastly Epicatechin (EC) which corresponds to approximately 6 % of total catechins (161).

When you have consumed green tea, the components of green tea can undergo metabolic processing like methylation, glucuronidation and sulphation which leads to the production of active metabolites. The positive health effects of green tea depend on the factors described above and the bioavailability after consumption.

All four types of catechins in green tea can be measured and detected in blood plasma but only EGC and EG can be detected in urine. Two hours after the consumption of green tea the top concentrations of blood plasma components occur, while after four to six hours after the consumption the top concentrations of urine components occur (161).

EGCG is the most common studied catechin of green tea that has several cancer related mechanisms which include DNA hypermetylation, inhibition of angiogenesis, telomerase activity, NF-kB, metastasis, tumor cell growth, promotion of tumor cell apoptosis and induction of tumor suppressor genes.

The mechanism of inhibition of angiogenesis is suggested by a decrease in peptide levels of VEGF (vascular endothelial growth factor) and RNA, but also by interfering with dimerization with VEFR2 (vascular endothelial growth factor receptor 2) on VEGF.

The mechanism of inhibition of carcinogens is by increasing the levels of GST-pi (glutathione-S transferase pi) which inhibit carcinogenic-induced DNA damage through catalyze detoxification reactions.

Green tea helps to reduce the risk of cancer such as cardiac, breast, esophagus, colorectal, lung, stomach, prostate, pancreas and ovarian cancer.

In a recent study, it was showed that the risk of developing breast cancer was lower when participants consumed more cups of tea (1 – 5 + cups of tea) than zero cups of tea.

It was also showed that green tea or dietary supplements of the four types of catechins in green tea mixed together in a supplement are more effective than only one catechin dietary supplement, for example, EGCG (161).

Green tea is also good for decreasing the risk of cardiovascular disease (CVD). CVD involves many factors such as oxidative stress, inflammation, lipid metabolism and platelet aggregation. A study conducted on green tea and CVD showed that it was a 28 % lower risk of death of CVD between those people who consumed less than three cups of tea a day and those who consumed more than ten cups of tea a day. Another study showed that it was a 14 % lower risk of death of CVD between those people who consumed less than one cup of tea a day and those who consumed more than five cups of tea a day (161).

It has also been proven in studies with green tea extract in Japan, that after 12 weeks, the participants had decreased blood pressure (6.5 %), decreased body fat (10 %) and decreased levels of LDL (2.6 %) which leads to decreased risk for CVD. It has also been proven that patients with diabetes reduced the levels of hemoglobin A1c (HbA1c) from 6.2 % to 6.0 %, reduced the levels of fasting blood glucose from 135 to 128.8 mg / dl in just two months.

It has also been proven that participants who consumed three cups of green tea a day reduced the risk of myocardial infarction death by 11 %. Participants who consumed more than 14 cups of green tea a week had 10 % of the total myocardial infarction deaths, participants who consumed around 14 cups of green tea a week had 11 % of myocardial infarction deaths and participants who didn't consume any cups of green tea a week had 14 % of total deaths caused by myocardial infarction. Consumption of EGCG by patients who has CVD resulted in a rapidly improvement of vascular endothelial function. It is also showed that 300 mg of EGCG resulted in an improved arm artery fluid-mediated dilation from 7.1 % to 8.6 % after two hours.

In a study, participants consumed either 89 mg / day of flavonoids, 251 mg / day of flavonoids or 532 mg / day of flavonoids. The total deaths caused by CVD in the group that consumed 89 mg was 8.6 %, in the group that consumed 251 mg it was 6.4 % and in the last group that consumed 532 mg it was 5.0 % (161).

Green tea is also helpful for preventing inflammation. Some anti-inflammatory mechanisms of green tea components are: Regulation of signaling and IL-6 synthesis, increased synthesis of anti-inflammatory cytokine IL-10, decreased levels of the proinflammatory cytokines TNF-alpha and IL-1, decreased expression of the chemokine receptor CCR2 and reduced synthesis of destructive matrix metalloproteinases through TNF-alpha induced phosphorylation of MAPK (mitogen activated protein kinases).

It has been proven that catechins in green tea downregulate many inflammatory cytokines, chemokines and inflammatory markers like: IL-1beta, IL-1alpha, IL-8, IL-6, CRP (C-reactive protein) and INF-gamma (interferon gamma).

Other studies show that consumption of EGCG or green tea results in an inhibition of inflammation by suppressing factors known to regulate neutrophil function like GM-CSF (granulocyte-macrophage colony stimulating factor), IL-2, IL-1beta and TNF-alpha.

Other studies show that consumption of catechins from green tea make it harder for neutrophils to migrate to infected sites through decreasing the number of CAMs (leukocyte endothelial cell adhesion molecules like VCAM-1, ICAM-1 and E-selection) which are expressed on the surface of the endothelial cell.

To make the neutrophils take another way away from the inflammation site leads to reduced inflammation.

Neutrophil function and migration are parts of the

inflammatory response which green tea is helpful to prevent (161).

Green tea is also helpful against oxidative stress in the body. Oxidative stress is related to CVD and inflammation and is a negative result of ROS (reactive oxygen species) which can cause chronic inflammation in the body by the induction of chemokines, inflammatory cytokines and proinflammatory transcription factors. Green tea catechins have an antioxidant effect through: inducing antioxidant enzymes, salivation of ROS and inhibit prooxidative enzymes and inhibit redox sensitive transcription factors. The catechins in green tea have been proven to increase levels of antioxidants, affect levels of ROS, increase TAC (TAS) and reduce levels of inflammatory agents (161).

It has also been proven in some studies that EGCG in green tea is helpful to prevent platelet aggregation through activation of ADP (adenosine diphosphate) which inhibits platelet activation. EGCG also suppressed p38 MAPK phosphorylation of HSP27 (heat shock protein 27) which will inhibit the platelets' release of pro-thrombotic content (33).

EGCG also reduces the risk of lipid metabolism by decreasing the levels of LDL, total cholesterol and blood pressure. But a new study showed that the catechins in green tea are integrated into LDL particles where they can reduce LDL oxidation. Catechins prevent oxidation of LDL by acting as hydrogen donors to alpha-tocopherol radicals and by radical capture (161).

When it comes to antimicrobial properties, the catechins in green tea affect a large amount of gram-negative and gram-positive aerobic bacteria, fungi, viruses, anaerobacteria and at least one parasite. The antimicrobial mechanisms of green tea are: inhibition of enzymes like (cysteine proteinases, ATP synthase, protein tyrosine kinase, DNA gyras), inhibition of bacterial fatty acid synthesis, damage to cell membranes of the bacteria and inhibition of efflux Pump activity. It has also been proved that green tea consumption leads to fewer flu symptoms and cold, fewer febrile diseases and fewer infections with influenza A or B (161).

Green tea promotes even oral health through its
antimicrobial activity against dandruff such as
Streptococcus mutans and anti-inflammatory properties.
Its antimicrobial activity is helpful against bad breath.
The effects of improved oral health caused by green tea is
through a reduction of caries and periodontist.
When it comes to caries, EGCG inhibits and binds
bacterial amylases and saliva (mainly alpha-amylase).
EGCG inhibits the function and transcription of LDH
which prevents the synthesis of acid from carbohydrates.
Caries is caused by a biofilm on the surface of the teeth
which is produced by oral bacteria like *Streptococcus
mutans*. EGCG inhibits the bacteria's ability to create an
acidic environment, reduces the production of biofilm
and inhibits the adhesion of bacteria to the teeth. An
increase in oral peroxidase activity has also been related
to consumption of green tea. EGCG also inhibits
hydrophobic interactions and hydrogen bonding of
bacterial collagenases.
When it comes to periodontitis (the tissues surrounding
the teeth get affected by inflammatory diseases which can

lead loss of teeth), EGCG inhibits the synthesis of IL-8 and matrix metalloproteins which both destroy tissue. EGCG also inactivates bacterial collagenases and inhibits the bacteria's ability to bind via fimbriae to epithelial cells in the mouth. Green tea is also effective against periodontal health when it comes to bleeding gums, dental bone erosion, assess to probe deep and fastening loss. Another effect of green tea is that it has been proven to prevent the progression and development of periodontitis and reduce dental loss (161).

The best tea to consume for the most health benefits is green tea but black tea is also good. In black tea, there is a group of teaflavins, more common named as teaflavin-3,3'-digallate (TF3) which is similar with the EGCG in green tea when it comes to the antioxidant activity. In a study, it was showed that a bag of green tea contained 165 mg of bile acid which is a form of phenols and a bag of black tea contained 124 mg of bile acid. It was also showed that green tea contained 436 mg of vitamin C equivalents (antioxidants) and black tea contained 239 mg of vitamin C equivalents (162).

Green tea contains about 24 – 40 mg of caffeine while a cup of coffee contains about 30 – 175 mg of caffeine depending on the concentration of the coffee.

An interesting thing about green tea is that in some studies, it was showed that men who consumed green tea during a workout lost 17 % more body fat than men who did not consume green tea during a workout. This means that you can lose more body fat percentage in the long term with green tea than without green tea.

In some studies, it has also been shown that EGCG can make the absorption of fat less effective due to inhibition of lipases in the small intestine. It has also been shown that the energy consumption in the liver increases of EGCG. Hot drinks like tea increases the temperature around the liver and in the core which results in reduced appetite. Reduced appetite and increased body temperature can also be achieved by theobromine and caffeine which both exists in tea. Therefore, intake of tea before a meal or during the phase when you are fasting make you consume less calories of the meal and make you satisfied earlier. Intake of tea before exercising, increases the tea's fat burning properties, and it also gives you more energy for the exercise. EGCG and caffeine together, increases the fat burning process of the fat in the abdomen and the subcutaneous fat. The caffeine makes this possible, because the caffeine makes the fat release from the fat cells (163,164).

Coffee

Coffee is a mix of chemicals where the main source is caffeine. Coffee also contains lipids, carbohydrates, vitamins, nitrogenous compounds, minerals, phenolic compounds and alkaloids. A cup of home-made coffee (150 ml) contains between 30 mg and 175 mg of caffeine depending on the concentration of the coffee. Caffeine works through antagonism of adenosine receptor, which is an endogenous inhibitory neuromodulator that calls for sleepiness. Caffeine stimulates its effects in the central nervous system. A caffeine intake of 300 mg/day or 2-3 cups of coffee a day leads to increased metabolism, increased blood pressure and diuresis. This intake of caffeine is not associated with side effects such as behavioral changes and cardiovascular stimulatory effects in healthy adults.

Women that are trying to become pregnant or is pregnant should not consume more than 300 mg of caffeine / day due it can harm the mother and the fetus because caffeine crosses human placenta and quickly increases the concentrations in the mother and the fetus. Caffeine has led to impaired fetal growth or spontaneous abortion. Children that consume too high concentrations of caffeine can develop behavioral changes like anxiety and nervousness, therefore the Federal Department of Health, Ottawa, Ontario recommends children to never ever consume more than 2.5 mg / kg body weight / day. This is the upper limit of caffeine consumption in children (165).

The coffee beans contain phenolic antioxidant compounds and the largest polyphenol in coffee is called chlorogenic acid (165). Reduced insulin secretion and slower increase of blood sugar due to delayed absorption of glucose in the small intestine are some effects of chlorogenic acid. Trigonelin, an alkaloid in coffee, also delays the absorption of glucose in the small intestine (166). The medium-roasted coffee contains the highest concentration of antioxidant activity (165).

Higher concentrations of LDL cholesterol and total serum cholesterol has been associated with coffee consumption. Two diterpenes in coffee oil is kahweol and cafestol. These two diterpenes are the major cholesterol enhancing compounds in coffee. These diterpenes are removed through paper filters and this means that unfiltered coffee contains much higher concentrations of diterpenes which lead to a higher increase in serum cholesterol than brewing coffee (165).

Coffee is also good for the health. Some studies have proven that coffee can prevent multiple chronic diseases. If coffee is consumed regularly it can help to decrease the risk of diabetes type 2, liver damage such as cirrhosis, hepatic injury and hepatocellular carcinoma, Parkinson's disease and Alzheimer's disease. Coffee can also help to improve the endurance performance when it comes to physical activity that lasts for a long time. It was also showed that suicide risks decreased with 13 % for every cup that was consumed daily. Coffee is also a good protector against cancer such as colorectal and liver cancer (165).

Coffee has also some cardiovascular effects like hypertension, tachycardia and sometimes arrhythmia. These effects may occur in people that are sensitive against coffee and those people that rarely drinks coffee (161). If your sleep affects negative from drinking coffee, then you should not consume coffee after 2 PM. You can drink the cups of coffee you need in the morning when you are fasting. There is also a very weak association between coffee and the risk of stroke, but more research needs on this subject (165).

An important factor of caffeine is that the calcium absorption in the gastrointestinal tract slightly decreases when caffeine is consumed. Because of this, it is very important that the vitamin D intake and calcium intake is high enough and a restriction of 2 – 3 cups of coffee per day would be a great spot to aim for to lower the risks of osteoporosis and its related fracture among the older generation of people (165).

Caffeine contains dopamine which results in reward effects in the brain, and dopamine is necessary for the human to feel good. Just like tea, coffee reduces appetite (167). The caffeine should be consumed from either tea or coffee if you want to be healthy and burn fat. The insulin sensitivity can be impaired if the caffeine is consumed from pills and energy drinks, an impaired insulin sensitivity can result in less effect of the fat burning process. Energy drinks that contain caffeine, also contain sugar which reduces the fat burning process and can result in impaired insulin sensitivity (166).

Alcohol

The recommended intake for men is less than 20 grams per day (approximately 2 units) or less than 5 % of the total energy intake per day and the recommended intake for women is less than 10 grams per day (approximately

1 unit) or less than 5 % of the total energy intake per day (168).

One gram of alcohol equals 7 calories which is higher than carbohydrates and protein but not higher than fat. In the small intestine in the body, the alcohol is efficiently absorbed through passive diffusion and the alcohol is distributed to the body's total water compartments. 95 % - 90 % of the absorbed alcohol is oxidized in the body and the rest (5 % - 10 %) is lost in the urine and through expired air.

It has been proven that the quality of the diet (decreased intake of fruits, dairy products and vegetables) can be impaired when the intake of alcohol is increased. Increased nutrient loss in the urine and impaired absorption of nutrients can be a result of a high intake of alcohol, even deficiencies in magnesium, ascorbic acid, phosphorus, thiamine, protein and vitamin D among high alcohol consumers, therefore, the intake of alcohol is recommended to a moderate level (168,169).

Alcohol affects all the body's organs in a toxic way and the damage of alcohol contributes to mortality and morbidity. The total amount of alcohol to which the body is exposed is a mainly determinant for the harmful health effects of alcohol. So, even in individuals who are not visibly drunk, the development of alcohol damage might occur. Alcohol-related damage to the body is likely to occur of 70 grams of alcohol intake per day (169).

The secretion of parathormone which decreases insulin sensitivity and inhibits fat burning is reduced by alcohol, which means that insulin sensitivity increases by alcohol. Increased insulin sensitivity leads to protection against diabetes type II and the weight becomes also more stabilized. Alcohol is also a good protection against cardiovascular disease. Adiponectin and glucagon which are fat burning hormones are increased by alcohol. Dopamine is also released by alcohol. There are 7 calories in one gram of alcohol, but around 3 calories of these 7 calories are lost through the transformation to heat when the alcohol goes to the liver.

In red wine, the content of antioxidants is high. Red wine contains a molecule called resveratrol, which in tests of human fat cells have been shown to inhibit the division of fat cells and the maturation of proadipocytes, which is the form that adipocytes have before they become adipocytes. Resveratrol might result in less fat cells in the body (170,171,172).

Alcohol, especially red wine, is good for weight loss, but the health benefits of red wine appears only when the recommendations above are followed. Intakes over the recommendations can lead to a toxic effect and a lot of calories which easily can result in an intake of calories that is higher than what the body expenditures, which leads to weight gain (173).

Alcohol related to body weight

No consistent association between alcohol intake and weight gain was showed in a review of 31 publications with four clinical trials and 13 prospective cohort studies. But in some studies that included over 2 – 3 drinks of alcohol per day showed an association with weight gain. According to the evidence, beer (about 2.5 – 6 volume %

of alcohol) and spirits (about 40 volume % of alcohol) is related to a higher weight gain than wine (about 12 volume % of alcohol). Currently, there are not enough of evidence on body weight and alcohol intake, and, therefore, no conclusion can be drawn right now (174).

1 unit equals 8 – 12 grams of alcohol and corresponds to one bottle of beer (330 mL), one glass of spirits (40 mL) or one glass of wine (120 mL). 2 units equals 16 – 24 grams of alcohol and corresponds to two bottles of beer (660 mL), two glasses of spirits (80 mL) or two glasses of wine (240 mL) (175).

Chapter 16

Research on training interventions for Weight Loss

Article 1 (176)

The weights should be low during the first two weeks of training because the patients' muscles will prevent muscle soreness and will adapt to the training but even so they can learn the techniques of the movements. The purpose with the training from the third week is hypertrophy which means that the patient should do three sets per muscle group three days per week with 10 – 15 repetitions per set without interruption until the patient can't lift the weight for more repetitions. When the patient can perform more than 15 reps per set, the weight should increase until the patient can perform 15 reps per set with the new weight. From now on, the patient should increase the sets per muscle group every four weeks until the patient performs a maximum of 10 sets per muscle group per week. The resistance program should consist of exercises for the biggest muscle groups. For the upper body, the patient can perform dumbbell flyes (for the breast), bench press (for the breast), pull downs (for the back), shoulder press (for the shoulders), triceps extensions and biceps curls (for the arms) and exercises for the core (abdominal muscles and lower back and the side of the abdominal). For the lower body, the patient can perform leg press (for the quadriceps femoris which is the front part of the upper leg) (176).

What shows the research of this type of training?

One study showed that lean body mass associated with the age progression was prevented and resting energy expenditure was increased due to increased muscle protein turnover when patients performed resistance training two times per week.

Another study included 35 overweight men who either was in a control group, a diet group performing aerobic endurance training, a diet group or a diet group that performed both resistance training and aerobic endurance training showed that after 12 weeks, the weight loss was significant and equal in the groups. This study showed that resistance training is good for avoiding catabolism of body protein which changes the relationship between fat mass and lean body mass.

In another study where 29 obese men either consumed a hypocaloric diet (consuming less calories than the body expenditures), consumed a hypocaloric diet in combination with resistance training or in combination with aerobic endurance training during 16 weeks showed that all the obese men lost 12.4 kg (27.55 lbs) and lost 9.7 kg (21.55 lbs) of total adipose tissue in all the groups.

Interesting was that lean body mass only was preserved when hypocaloric diet was combined with training.

A further study showed that resistance training two times per week for 39 weeks didn't result in any significant weight loss, but instead, the patients lost 0.98 kg (2.17 lbs) of fat mass, increased 0.89 kg (1.97 lbs) in more lean body mass than the control group and lost 1.63 % more body fat than the control group.

In another study where participants performed resistance training three times per week showed that the participants lost 13.05 % more body fat, increased 5.05 % more lean body mass and lost 12.11 % more fat mass than the control group (176).

There are also some studies made on visceral adipose tissue. Adipose tissue is a huge endocrine organ that secretes substances like leptin, adiponectin, tumor necrosis factor alpha, resistin, plasminogen activator inhibitor-1 and interleukin 6. Too much of visceral adipose tissue is connected with the development of hypertension, type 2 diabetes, dyslipidemia, insulin resistance and cardiovascular diseases (176).

A lot of studies show positive results of resistance training on visceral adipose tissue, for example, a study made by Treuth et al. showed decreased visceral fat in older women and men after resistance training for 16 weeks.

In two studies made by Ross et al. where middle-aged obese men either consumed a hypocaloric diet, consumed a hypocaloric diet combined with resistance training (70 % to 80 % of 1RM – when you can only perform one repetition with the weight you are using) or consumed a hypocaloric diet combined with aerobic endurance training showed that visceral fat loss was similar between the diets combined with resistance training and aerobic endurance training. In a follow-up study by Ross et al. it was showed that 32 % of visceral fat was lost in the diet group without training, 39 % of visceral fat was lost in the diet combined with aerobic endurance training and 40 % of visceral fat was lost in the diet combined with resistance training group.

The research shows a positive correlation between visceral fat reduction and resistance training and therefore Ross et al. recommend resistance training combined with a hypocaloric diet for obese individuals who want to reduce the visceral adipose tissue (176).

The conclusions of this article are that resistance training, with or without a hypocaloric diet, can increase muscular strength, increase lean body mass, increase resting metabolic rate, reduce subcutaneous adipose tissue in the abdominal region and reduce visceral fat in both obese women and men (176).

Article 2 (177)
Different types of training (review)
In this article, the authors have described many articles based on if the participants followed training programs and diets. The results are also revealed. I will describe these articles shortly now.

In the first study by Castaneda et al. where 31 participants followed a resistance training program included 8 reps with 60 – 80 % of 1RM, three times per week resulted in increased lean body mass.

In the second study by Cauza et al. where 17 participants followed an aerobic endurance training program included 60 % of VO2max, three times per week resulted in decreased body fat percentage, decreased fat mass and decreased total fat. In the same study where 22 participants followed a resistance program included 10 – 15 reps or fatigue three times per week resulted in decreased body fat percentage, decreased fat mass, decreased total fat and increased lean body mass (177).

In the third study by Dunstan et al. where 16 participants followed a resistance training program included 8 – 10 reps with 50 – 85 % of 1RM resulted in decreased body fat, decreased waist circumference and decreased body weight (177).

In the fourth study by Irving et al. where 9 participants followed a high intensity program included a rating of perceived exertion of 15 – 17 (very intense) three times per week and rating of perceived exertion of 10 – 12 (medium intense) two times per week with a total of 5 times per week resulted in decreased waist circumference, decreased amount of abdominal (visceral, subcutaneous) fat, decreased fat mass, decreased body weight and decreased BMI (177).

In the fifth study by Sigal et al. where 60 participants followed an aerobic endurance training program included 60 – 75 % of VO2max three times per week resulted in decreased abdominal subcutaneous fat, decreased fat mass, decreased waist circumference, decreased body weight and decreased BMI.
In the same study by Sigal et al. where 64 participants followed a resistance training program included 7 – 9 reps to fatigue three times per week resulted in decreased abdominal subcutaneous fat and decreased waist circumference (177).

In the sixth and last study by Stewart et al. where 51 participants followed a resistance training program included 10 – 15 reps (50 % of 1RM) three times per week resulted in decreased abdominal subcutaneous and visceral fat, decreased body fat percentage, decreased waist circumference, decreased body weight, decreased BMI and increased lean body mass (177).

Studies on resistance training for weight loss

There are few studies that have analyzed the connection between resistance training and weight loss. In a study where participants followed a 15 % (12 kg – 26.6 lbs) diet-induced weight loss combined with resistance training increased the insulin sensitivity with 49 % and lost visceral fat with 37 %. The participants who combined diet with resistance training lost 29 % more body weight than the participants (women) who lost 15 % of their body weight without training. In a follow-up study, participants who combined diet with resistance training did not regain the visceral fat they had lost, but participants who did not exercise regained over 70 % of the lost visceral fat. The obese participants who combined diet with resistance training also showed a lower regain of total body fat compared with the participants who did only diet (177).

Article 3 (178)

In a study by Lopes et al. 33 girls in the age between 13 –
17 years old were assigned into three groups. The first
group included overweight training and consisted of 15
participants and the second group included overweight
control and consisted of 16 participants and the last group
included normal-weight group and consisted of 15
participants. All the groups performed the same training
program. The training program consisted of a
combination of resistance training and aerobic training in
the same session. The resistance program consisted of six
exercises which were leg extension, leg press, bench
press, leg curl, arm curl and lateral pull-down and the
aerobic training consisted of walking/running with an
intensity of 50 – 85 % of VO2max during 30 minutes.
For the first four weeks, the participants would perform
10 reps for 3 sets for each exercise and rest 1 minute
between the sets. During week four to eight, the
participants would perform 8 reps for 3 sets for each
exercise and rest 1.5 minutes between the sets. During
week eight to twelve, the participants would perform 6
reps for 3 sets for each exercise and rest 1.5 – 2 minutes

between the sets. The workloads for the upper body would be increased with 0.5 kg (1.1 lbs) and 1 kg (2.22 lbs) for lower body every new week. So, if the participants performed, let's say, 20 kg (44.4 lbs) for leg curls the entire first week, then the second week, the participants would perform 21 kg (46.6 lbs) for leg curls. This type of training program was created in the way that the participants would perform the resistance training first for approximately 30 minutes and then the aerobic training for approximately 30 minutes in the same session during approximately 60 minutes three times a week during 12 weeks (178).

The results of this type of training
The body weight increased in the overweight training group from 77.4 kg (172 lbs) ± 12.3 kg (27.33 lbs) to 77.6 kg (172.44 lbs) ± 12.7 kg (28.22 lbs) and the body weight also increased in the overweight control group from 75.2 kg (167.11 lbs) ± 12.0 kg (26.66 lbs) to 76.3 kg (169.55 lbs) after the 12 weeks of training without a specific diet plan.

The body fat percentage decreased in the overweight training group from 45.2 % ± 4.8 % to 43.5 % ± 4.6 % while the body fat percentage increased in the overweight control group from 45.4 % ± 5.9 % to 46.0 % ± 6.3 % after the 12 weeks of training without a specific diet plan. The body fat in kg (lbs) decreased in the overweight training group due the percentage of the body fat decreased, but the numbers were as followed, 33.6 kg (74.66 lbs) ± 8.0 kg (17.77 lbs) to 32.5 kg (72.22 lbs) ± 8.2 kg (18.22 lbs). In the overweight control group, the body fat in kg (lbs) increased from 32.9 kg (73.11 lbs) ± 9.3 kg (20.66 lbs) to 33.6 kg (74.66 lbs) ± 10.0 kg (22.22 lbs) after the 12 weeks of training.

Fat-free mass increased in the overweight training group from 39.9 kg (88.66 lbs) ± 5.0 kg (11.11 lbs) to 41.3 kg (91.77 lbs) ± 4.8 kg (10.66 lbs). The fat-free mass decreased in the overweight control group from 38.3 kg (85.11 lbs) ± 3.7 kg (8.22 lbs) to 38.1 kg (84.66 lbs) ± 4.1 kg (9.11 lbs).

The leg press increased in the overweight training group from 164.7 kg (366 lbs) ± 33.9 kg (75.33 lbs) to 212.4 kg

(472 lbs), it also increased in the overweight control group from 166.3 kg (369.55 lbs) ± 33.6 kg (74.66 lbs) to 179.7 kg (399.33 lbs) ± 31.0 kg (68.88 lbs).

The bench press increased in the overweight training group from 30.0 kg (66.6 lbs) ± 4.6 kg (10.22 lbs) to 37.4 kg (83.11 lbs) ± 5.6 kg (12.44 lbs), it also increased in the overweight control group from 30.5 kg (67.77 lbs) ± 4.0 kg (8.88 lbs) to 31.2 kg (69.33 lbs) ± 4.2 kg (9.33 lbs). Lastly, the VO2max increased in the overweight training group from 30.2 ml/kg/min ± 3.4 ml/kg/min to 35.2 ml/kg/min ± 2.4 ml/kg/min, it also increased in the overweight control group from 30.9 ml/kg/min ± 3.9 ml/kg/min to 32.1 ml/kg/min ± 4.5 ml/kg/min (178).

The two different groups had almost the same results, but the results were always a little better in the group that exercised which shows us that exercising without any specific diet is more beneficial to us than only diet without exercising.

Article 4 (179)

In this study, 97 participants in the age between 40 to 66 years old performed either aerobic exercise, resistance exercise or combination exercise for 12 weeks. The aerobic exercise should follow the regimen of 30 minutes of treadmill walking at 60 % of heart rate maximum five days per week. To estimate the heart rate maximum, the Karvonen equation was done (220 − age = maximum heart rate, then you take that number times 0.60 and you get 60 % of heart rate maximum). The resistance exercise should follow the regimen of 30 minutes five days per week with four sets of 8 − 12 repetitions at 10 RM for leg curl, bench press, leg press, rear deltoid row and leg extension where the sets should be completed in around 30 seconds with 1 minute rest between sets. The combination exercise should follow the regimen of 15 minutes of aerobic exercise (treadmill walking at 60 % of heart rate maximum) and 15 minutes of resistance exercise where the same exercises would be performed as described above but with two sets of each exercise instead of four sets. To get the right workloads of 10 reps per exercise, the participants started by trying some workloads and if they could perform more than 10 reps per set then the workload was increased until only 10 reps could be performed during the 2 or 4 sets.

The first two weeks of the training program, the participants exercised for three days per week and after two weeks, the participants exercised five days per week. The participants could perform the exercises at home if they wanted. At home, the participants would perform resistance exercise included of lunges, biceps curls, calf lift, dumbbell raise and triceps extension with three sets of 10 reps while the combination group performed lunges and biceps curls for two sets and calf lift, dumbbell raise, triceps extension, push-ups, back extension and sit ups for 2 sets. When the participants could perform more than 12 reps per set, the workload would be increased with 2.5 kg (5.55 lbs).

The energy intake was set at 2087 ± 251 calories with 42.5 ± 3.1 % carbohydrates of the total energy intake, 18.3 ± 1.3 % protein of the total energy intake and 35.2 ± 2.6 % fat of the total energy intake for the first 8 weeks in the aerobic group. From week 8 to 11, the energy intake was set at 1784 ± 168 calories with $44.4 \pm 2.6 \%$ carbohydrates of the total energy intake, $19.7 \pm 1.4 \%$ protein of the total energy intake and $33.1 \pm 1.9 \%$ fat of the total energy intake and for the 12:th week, the energy intake was set at 1714 ± 119 calories with $41.2 \pm 2.3 \%$ carbohydrates of the total energy intake, $20.8 \pm 1.4 \%$ protein of the total energy intake and $35.1 \pm 1.8 \%$ fat of the total energy intake in the aerobic group (179).

The energy intake was set at 1857 ± 99 calories with $40.2 \pm 1.6 \%$ carbohydrates of the total energy intake, $19.8 \pm 1.1 \%$ protein of the total energy intake and $36.0 \pm 1.2 \%$ fat of the total energy intake for the first 8 weeks in the resistance group. From week 8 to 11, the energy intake was set at 1727 ± 114 calories with $41.7 \pm 1.9 \%$ carbohydrates of the total energy intake, $19.0 \pm 0.7 \%$ protein of the total energy intake and $34.8 \pm 1.8 \%$ fat of the total energy intake and for the 12:th week, the energy intake was set at 1656 ± 112 calories with $39.4 \pm 2.0 \%$ carbohydrates of the total energy intake, $20.2 \pm 1.0 \%$

protein of the total energy intake and 36.4 ± 1.4 % fat of the total energy intake in the resistance group (179).

The energy intake was set at 1833 ± 77 calories with 44.2 ± 1.9 % carbohydrates of the total energy intake, 19.1 ± 0.9 % protein of the total energy intake and 33.9 ± 1.7 % fat of the total energy intake for the first 8 weeks in the combination group. From week 8 to 11, the energy intake was set at 1845 ± 102 calories with 44.8 ± 1.9 % carbohydrates of the total energy intake, 18.5 ± 1.0 % protein of the total energy intake and 35.7 ± 1.7 % fat of the total energy intake and for the 12:th week, the energy intake was set at 1652 ± 96 calories with 43.4 ± 1.9 % carbohydrates of the total energy intake, 18.4 ± 1.1 % protein of the total energy intake and 35.7 ± 1.4 % fat of the total energy intake in the combination group (179).

The results of this type of training and diet
In the aerobic group, the body weight decreased from 91.9 kg (204.22 lbs) ± 4.1 kg (9.11 lbs) to 91.0 kg (202.22 lbs) ± 4.0 kg (8.88 lbs) in twelve weeks. The

body fat percentage in the aerobic group decreased from 44.6 % ± 1.9 % to 44.1 % ± 1.8 % in twelve weeks (179).

In the resistance group, the body weight decreased from 89.3 kg (198.44 lbs) ± 4.5 kg (10 lbs) to 89.2 kg (198.22 lbs) ± 4.4 kg (9.77 lbs) in twelve weeks. The body fat percentage in the resistance group decreased from 43.7 % ± 1.3 % to 43.2 % ± 1.4 % in twelve weeks (179).

In the combination group, the body weight decreased from 90.0 kg (200 lbs) ± 4.0 kg (8.88 lbs) to 88.4 kg (196.44 lbs) ± 3.6 kg (8 lbs) in twelve weeks. The body fat percentage in the combination group decreased from 45.8 % ± 1.6 % to 44.8 % ± 1.8 % in twelve weeks (179).

This study showed that the combination exercise had the greatest weight loss and reduction of the body fat percentage among these three groups.

Article 5 (180)

In this study, 196 participants in the age between 18 – 70 years old with a BMI over 30 kg/m² performed either resistance training, aerobic training or combination training for 8 – 10 weeks. The resistance training included 8 exercises with 8 – 12 repetitions for 3 sets 3 days per week. In the aerobic training group, the participants would reach 19.2 km/week (around 12 miles/week) with an intensity of 75 % of VO2max on an elliptical trainer, treadmill or cycle ergometer. The combination training consisted of the resistance training and the aerobic training mixed together, where the aerobic training was performed first followed by the resistance training. The duration of the workouts wouldn't exceed 60 minutes (180).

In the resistance group, for the first 1 – 2 weeks, the participants would perform 1 set per exercise, for the third and fourth week, the participants would perform two sets per exercise and after the fifth week, the participants would perform three sets per exercise. The workloads were increased with 5 lbs (2.25 kg) every time the participants performed three sets of 12 reps on two of three days per week (180).

The results of this type of training

The body weight in the resistance training group increased from 88.8 kg (197.33 lbs) to 89.61 kg (199.133 lbs). The body weight in the aerobic training group decreased from 88.8 kg (197.33 lbs) to 87.17 kg (193.711 lbs). The body weight in the combination training group decreased from 91.7 kg (203.77 lbs) to 90.06 kg (200.133 lbs). The greatest weight loss was, even here, in the combination training group (180).

The fat mass in the resistance training group decreased from 25.1 kg (55.77 lbs) to 24.88 kg (55.28 lbs). The fat mass in the aerobic training group decreased from 26.7 kg (59.33 lbs) to 25.45 kg (56.55 lbs). The fat mass in the combination training group decreased from 27.3 kg (60.66 lbs) to 25.41 kg (56.46 lbs). Even here, the greatest fat loss, was in the combination training group (180).

The lean body mass in the resistance group increased from 63.6 kg (141.33 lbs) to 64.64 kg (143.64 lbs). The lean body mass in the aerobic training group decreased from 61.0 kg (135.55 lbs) to 60.67 kg (134.82 lbs). The lean body mass in the combination training group increased from 62.8 kg (139.55 lbs) to 63.11 kg (140.24 lbs). The greatest increase in the lean body mass was here in the resistance training group, but the combination training group had greater increase in lean body mass than the aerobic training group (180).

Article 6 (181)

In this study, 83 overweight/obese sedentary women and men with the age between 55 years old ± 8.4 years old with a BMI of 35.3 ± 4.5 kg/m², followed either a resistance training program combined with a high or low protein rich diet, or followed no training program combined with a high or low protein rich diet for 16 weeks. Out of all these 83 participants, 59 participants completed the study.

The low-protein diet was set to around 1433 calories for women and around 1672 calories for men with 53 %

carbohydrates of the total energy intake, 26 % fat and 19 % protein. The high-protein diet was set to the same energy intake as in the low-protein diet but with 43 % carbohydrates, 22 % fat and 33 % protein of the total energy intake (181).

The resistance training program that the participants followed consisted of eight separate exercises (chest press, lat pull down, knee extension, leg press, shoulder press, triceps press, seated row and sit-ups). All these exercises were performed with machines except for the sit-ups. The exercises would be performed with 8 – 12 reps of 1 RM with two sets per exercise with 1 – 2 minutes of rest between sets. When the participants could perform two sets with over 12 reps, the workloads were increased until the participants could perform over 12 reps with the new workloads. The training sessions lasted for around 45 minutes three times per week on nonconsecutive days (Monday, Wednesday, Friday or Tuesday, Thursday, Saturday or, Wednesday, Friday, Sunday) (181).

The results of this type of training

The body weight in the low-protein group without resistance training decreased from 97.0 kg (215.55 lbs) ± 10.6 kg (23.55 lbs) to 88.4 kg (196.44 lbs) ± 11.2 kg (24.88 lbs). The body weight in the high-protein group without resistance training decreased from 102.7 kg (228.22 lbs) ± 15.4 kg (34.22 lbs) to 93.7 kg (208.22 lbs) ± 13.8 kg (30.66 lbs). The body weight in the low-protein group combined with resistance training decreased from 105.0 kg (233.33 lbs) ± 15.3 kg (34 lbs) to 94.5 kg (210 lbs) ± 15.4 kg (34.22 lbs). The body weight in the high-protein group combined with resistance training decreased from 107.6 kg (239.11 lbs) ± 15.5 kg (34.44 lbs) to 93.8 kg (208 lbs) ± 13.5 kg (30 lbs) in 16 weeks. The greatest weight loss was in the high-protein group combined with resistance training. That group lost 13.8 kg (30.66 lbs) ± 6.0 kg (13.33 lbs) (181).

The total body fat mass in the low-protein group without resistance training decreased from 38.5 kg (85.55 lbs) ± 8.0 kg (17.77 lbs) to 32.1 kg (71.33 lbs) ± 9.5 kg (21.11

lbs). The total body fat mass in the high-protein group without resistance training decreased from 40.4 kg (89.77 lbs) ± 8.4 kg (18.66 lbs) to 33.2 kg (73.77 lbs) ± 6.9 kg (15.33 lbs). The total body fat mass in the low-protein group combined with resistance training decreased from 40.4 kg (89.77 lbs) ± 10.0 kg (22.22 lbs) to 32.3 kg (71.77 lbs) ± 10.7 kg (23.77 lbs). The total body fat mass in the high-protein group combined with resistance training decreased from 42.9 kg (95.33 lbs) ± 11.6 kg (25.77 lbs) to 31.5 kg (70 lbs) ± 11.6 kg (25.77 lbs) in 16 weeks.

The greatest loss of total body fat mass was in the high-protein group combined with resistance training. That group lost 11.4 kg (25.33 lbs) ± 3.9 kg (8.66 lbs) in 16 weeks (181).

Article 7 (182)

In this study, 30 participants with a BMI over 30 kg/m² in the age between 20 and 40 years old followed either an aerobic training program or no training program at all. The training program started with warm up for 5 to 10 minutes followed by 20 to 40 minutes of submaximal intensity (220 – the age (25 for example) times 0.55 to 0.69 (55 % - 69 % of maximum heart rate). The participants would maintain this heart rate through the workout (20 to 40 minutes on the treadmill). When the participants were finished with the aerobic training, they would cool down for 5 to 10 minutes with slow and stretching activities (182).

The results of this type of training

The only relevant information in this study was the result of the BMI. In the group without aerobic training, the BMI decreased from 36 kg/m^2 to 35 kg/m^2 in 12 weeks (3 months). In the group with aerobic training included, the BMI decreased from 34.8 kg/m^2 to 33 kg/m^2 in 12 weeks (182).

This shows that aerobic training is beneficial for weight loss.

Article 8 (183)

In this study, 119 sedentary, obese or overweight adults followed either a resistance training program, an aerobic training program or a combination training program of resistance training and aerobic training. The resistance training included 8 – 12 reps with 3 sets per exercise 3 days per week. The aerobic training program included that the participants would reach around 12 miles (around 19 km) per week with an intensity of 65 % - 80 % of VO2max. The combination training program included 8 – 12 reps with 3 sets per exercise 3 days per week combined with 12 miles (19 km) per week with an intensity of 65 % - 80 % of VO2max.

In the resistance training group, the participants would perform one set during week 1 and 2, two sets during week 3 and 4 and three sets from week 5 to 8 to 10. Every time the participants could perform 12 reps for 3 sets for a specific exercise, the workloads would increase with 5 lbs (2.25 kg) until the participants could perform 12 reps for 3 sets again.

The food intake in the resistance training group was calculated to 2,009 calories per day. The food intake in the aerobic training group was calculated to 2,100 calories per day and in the combination training group, the food intake was calculated to 2,009 calories per day (183).

The results of this type of training

The body weight in the resistance training group increased with 0.83 kg (1.84 lbs) from 88.7 kg (197.11 lbs). The body weight in the aerobic training group decreased with 1.76 kg (3.91 lbs) from 88.0 kg (195.5 lbs). The body weight in the combination training group decreased with 1.63 kg (3.62 lbs) from 88.9 kg (197.5 lbs) (183).

The lean body mass in the resistance training group increased with 1.09 kg (2.42 lbs) from 54.4 kg (120.88 lbs). The lean body mass in the aerobic training group decreased with 0.10 kg (0.22 lbs) from 53.3 kg (118.44 lbs). The lean body mass in the combination training group increased with 0.81 kg (1.8 lbs) from 54.0 kg (120 lbs) (183).

The fat percentage in the resistance training group decreased with 0.65 % from 38.8 %. The fat percentage in the aerobic training group decreased with 1.01 % from 39.4 %. The fat percentage in the combination training group decreased with 2.04 % from 39.2 % (183).

This study showed that the aerobic training group had the greatest weight loss, the resistance training group had the greatest gain of lean body mass, while the combination training group had the greatest fat loss in percentage (183).

Article 9 (184)

In this study, 40 obese women with a body fat percentage of 47 % ± 1 % in the age between 62 years old ± 1 year old followed a weight loss hypocaloric diet and walking intervention. The participants would consume 250 – 350 calories per day during their maintenance levels for six months. Besides the diet, the participants would walk three days per week with an intensity of 50 – 60 % of the maximal heart rate for 30 – 45 minutes per walk. The participants walked two days on their own for 30 – 45 minutes and one day at the exercise facility under the supervision of an exercise physiologist (184).

The results of this type of training

The participants lost 6 kg (13.33 lbs) ± 1 kg (2.22 lbs) in six months with the starting body weight of 81 kg (180 lbs) ± 2 kg (4.44 lbs).

The participants lost 4 % ± 1 % of body fat percentage in six months with the starting body fat percentage of 47 % ± 1 % (184).

Article 10 (185)

An increased fat metabolism could reduce type II diabetes and obesity symptoms. Intensities between 47 % and 52 % of VO2max are the peak rates of fat oxidation of many people in general population. The fat oxidation is higher when persons are running instead of cycling. The rate of fat oxidation is slower if carbohydrates are ingested the hours before the exercise compared when persons are exercising in the fasted state. A fast over six hours increases fat oxidation. The rate of fat oxidation also decreases when high-fat diets are followed due to adaptations at the muscle level and decreased stores of glycogen (185).

Fasting compared to not fasting before endurance training on fat oxidation

In this part of the chapter, I will review three articles about exercising in the fasted state compared to the non-fasted state regarding free fatty acids. I used these articles for my examination project work, so they are by high value.

Article 11 (186)

In this study, participants would perform two 90-minute and two 60-minute cycle passes per week for six weeks with an intensity of 70 % of VO2max. The participants would either fast (no breakfast) before the workouts or consume a breakfast consisted of 646 – 907 calories before the workouts with maltodextrin during the workouts (185).

The results of this study

The fasted group had in average 388 ± 70 micromol/L free fatty acids in the beginning of the test and ended up with 1657 ± 136 micromol/L free fatty acids during the post-test. The no-fasted group had in average 418 ± 40 micromol/L free fatty acids in the beginning of the test and ended up with 1857 ± 132 micromol/L free fatty acids during the post-test (185).

This study indicated that the participants in the fasted state group had lower concentrations of free fatty acids in the post-test in this study which is beneficial for weight loss (185).

Article 12 (187)

In this study, participants would perform two 90-minute and two 60-minute cycling and running passes per week for six weeks with an intensity of 70 – 75 % of VO2max for the cycling workouts and 85 % of VO2max for the running workouts. The participants would either fast (no breakfast) before the workouts or consume a breakfast consisted of 675 calories before the workouts with maltodextrin during the workouts (186).

The results of this study

During the pre-test, the fasted group had in average 531 ± 54 micromol/L free fatty acids and in the post-test the fasted group had in average 305 ± 46 micromol/L free fatty acids. The no-fasted group had in the pre-test in average 481 ± 42 micromol/L free fatty acids and in the post-test in average 330 ± 46 micromol/L (186).

This study showed that the participants in the fasted group reached the lowest concentrations of free fatty acids in the post-test (186).

Article 13 (188)

In this study, participants would perform a cycling workout on a bike ergometer with a workload of 178 ± 8 watts with and intensity of 75 % of VO2max for 120 minutes on a pre-test and a post-test with three weeks apart. The participants would either fast (no breakfast) before the workouts or consume a carbohydrate-rich breakfast consisted of 722 calories before the workouts with maltodextrin during the exercise sessions (187).

The results of this study

During the pre-test, the fasted group had in average 358 ± 113 micromol per kg dry bodyweight of free fatty acids and four hours of resting after the post-test the fasted group had in average 44 ± 18 micromol per kg dry bodyweight of free fatty acids. During the pre-test, the no-fasted group had in average 57 ± 9 micromol per kg dry bodyweight of free fatty acids and four hours of resting after the post-test the no-fasted group had in average 34 ± 15 micromol per kg dry bodyweight of free fatty acids (187).

This study showed that the participants who consumed a carbohydrate-rich breakfast before the tests achieved the lowest concentrations of free fatty acids, but the fasted group achieved the highest difference in the concentration of free fatty acids (187).

Chapter 17

The original training program

This training program will be constructed as a progressively combination training program (combined aerobic endurance training with resistance training) since the research shows that combination training is the greatest training method for fat loss. With progressively, I mean that the training will increase in intensity when you develop more strength and fitness. This means that the workloads will increase and that the aerobic endurance workouts will become more intense than in the beginning. You will stick to the program until you have reached your goal body weight or your goal body fat percentage.

I will write the names of the exercises and I will explain how to do them with proper form so you avoid getting injured in the Appendix below. When you have read how to do the exercises and you feel like you still don't know how to perform the exercises, many gyms have personal trainers who give you an introduction of how the exercises will be done for free when you sign up to the gym. You can send me an email and I will describe more how the exercises will be performed. But, I think you understand how to perform them after you have read the explanations in the Appendix below. When you will perform the exercises for the first time, it is very IMPORTANT that you take it slow and start with a low weight on the exercises for reducing the risk of injury. It is also important that you start of slow on the aerobic endurance exercises for reducing the risk of injury.

The exercises for the resistance training

The major exercises we will focus on and become strong at are the following: Bench Press (Machine), Lat Pull Downs (Machine), Shoulder Press (Machine), Lateral Raises (Machine), Biceps Curls (Machine), Triceps extensions (Machine), Leg Press (Machine), and Calves Press (Machine).

These are the exercises for the resistance training that we are going to focus on.

The exercises for the core that we will focus on are the following: Sit-Ups, Side-to-Sides and Back Extensions.

Here are all the exercises that we will focus on for the resistance training.

The goal here is to perform 8 – 12 reps for 1 set per exercise with a rest time of 30 seconds between sets. But, this is the goal we will aim for, so to reach this goal we must progress to reach it. Therefore, I will below, describe what you will do for the first weeks until you can follow this plan.

You will perform the resistance training three days per week.

The aerobic endurance training

For the aerobic endurance training, we will perform different types of exercises. The exercises you will perform are, either, walking (outside or on a treadmill), cycling (outside or at a spinning cycle), running (outside or on a treadmill), rowing (machine), swimming, cross-training (on a cross-trainer), dancing etc. We will perform the aerobic training for at least 30 minutes in the beginning and then progressively increase the speed or the distance for the workout. The longer you exercise the more calories you burn. You will burn most of the calories during the aerobic exercises and it is also from this type of training the fat oxidation will be increased.

You will perform the aerobic training at the same days as the resistance training, but it is recommended that you perform aerobic exercises every day.

Week 1

This is your first training week and here we will perform 1 set per exercise for 8 – 12 reps three days per week. We will do this for minimizing the risk of injury and burnout. We will also do this for neuronal adaptation in the muscles and for learning the techniques of the exercises. For the aerobic training, during the first week, we will start slowly by performing 30 minutes of aerobic training per day.

Week 2

For the second week, we will still perform 1 set per exercise for 8 – 12 reps three days per week combined with 30 minutes of aerobic training per day. When you perform the aerobic training this week, you will either increase the speed, so that you walk/run/swim/row/cycle faster than the last week or you will increase the distance. You have now get used to the resistance exercises, so now you will only try to progress with a proper form.

Week 3 and forward

For the third week and forward we will perform 1 set per exercise for 8 – 12 reps three days per week. We will combine this with 30 minutes of aerobic training and progressively increase, either, the speed or the distance of the workout. If you feel like you want to build more muscles, then you can perform 2 sets per exercise instead of 1 set per exercise. If you add 1 extra set per exercise your training session will be prolonged with around 20 minutes, and as a beginner, I think that those 20 extra minutes are not worth it, because you will become burned out and tired of going to the gym. So, you can add that extra set per exercise when you have lost some body weight and feel like you have more energy to workout. But, remember, that this is not a bodybuilding program, it is a program for people who wants to lose body weight and become healthy. You can focus on building more muscles when you have reached your goal body weight and then want to become stronger. But for now, just focus on the weight loss and 1 set per exercise and you'll be fine.

Below, I will write the training program that you will follow.

Week 1

You will always perform the resistance training first when you will train both resistance training and aerobic training at the same days, because exercising on a fasted stomach increases the fat oxidation more than exercising on a no-fasted stomach, accordingly to the research above.

The exercises for week 1

Monday

- **Bench Press (Machine) – 8 – 12 reps for 1 set.**
- **Lat Pull Downs (Machine) – 8 – 12 reps for 1 set.**
- **Shoulder Press (Machine) – 8 – 12 reps for 1 set.**
- **Lateral Raises (Machine) – 8 – 12 reps for 1 set.**
- **Biceps Curls (Machine) – 8 – 12 reps for 1 set.**
- **Triceps Extensions (Machine) – 8 – 12 reps for 1 set.**
- **Leg Press (Machine) – 8 – 12 reps for 1 set.**
- **Calves Press (Machine) – 8 – 12 reps for 1 set.**
- **Sit-Ups (Machine) – 8 – 12 reps for 1 set.**
- **Side-to-Sides (Machine) – 8 – 12 reps for 1 set.**
- **Back Extensions (Machine) – 8 – 12 reps for 1 set.**

Combined with aerobic training

- **30 – 60 minutes of walking/running/cycling/rowing/swimming/cro** ss-training with an intensity of 47 % and 52 % of VO2max. If you have an intensity over 52 % of VO2max, it doesn't matter that much, as long as you do your exercise. The intensity of 47 % - 52 % of VO2max is the peak rate of fat oxidation, and if you, for example, have an intensity of 75 % of VO2max, you will only have a decreased rate of fat oxidation but you will burn more calories.

Notes on the workout

In the beginning of every training session, you will warm up for 5 – 15 minutes to get warmer and reduce the risk of injury, because when you exercise with cold muscles, the risk of injury is very high. The warm up will consist of walking in a very slow pace on a treadmill, or workout in a very slow pace on a cross-trainer just to increase the blood flow to the muscles. This is your first week of training and therefore you will start with low intensity on the resistance training with 1 set per exercise. It is better to pick a weight that is lower, so you can perform the exercises with a proper form and reduce the risk of injury. Between the exercises, you will rest for 30 seconds.

When you will perform the aerobic training, you will have an intensity of 47 % - 52 % of VO2max. You can calculate your VO2max in two ways. The first way is to take 220 (minus) – your age (for example, 38) which is 182. This is not your real VO2max, but it is a good way of estimating your VO2max. 47 – 52 % of VO2max is calculated by taking 182 (times) x 0.47 or 0.52 which is 85.5 – 94.6 beats per minute (BPM).

The other way to calculate your VO2max is by taking 208 (minus) – (0.7 x age). First you calculate 0.7 x age (for example 38) which is 26.6, then you take 208 – 26.6 which is 181.4 BPM. To calculate 47 – 52 % of VO2max, you do the same thing as in the example above which is by taking 181.4 x 0.47 or 0.52 which is 85 – 94 BPM.

So, how do you know that you have an intensity of 47 – 52 % during your workout? On many treadmills and spinning cycles, there are sensors on the hand grips that measure your heart rate. The heart rate from the sensors on the hand grips on the machines isn't your true heart rate, because normally, there is a difference between ±5 – 10 BPM from your real heart rate, but they can be used anyway. If you place your hands on those sensors, you will automatically see your heart rate.

The other way is by buying a watch or pulse band that measures your heart rate (for example a fit bit).

At the end of every training session, you will cool down by walking in a very slow pace on a treadmill or cross-trainer for 5 – 15 minutes just to shake off the muscle groups you have been training. You can stretch the muscle groups if you want to after every training session.

Tuesday

On this day, you will only perform aerobic training. For example, you can walk for 30 – 60 minutes, you can run for 30 – 60 minutes or spinning for 30 – 60 minutes in whatever pace you want, but try to hit at least 47 % - 52 % of your VO2max. Try to do some aerobic exercises on the days. Personally, I go for a long walk for 60 +

minutes or go for a run for $30 - 60 +$ minutes just to do some activity and reduce the sedentary.

Wednesday

- **Bench Press (Machine) – 8 – 12 reps for 1 set.**
- **Lat Pull Downs (Machine) – 8 – 12 reps for 1 set.**
- **Shoulder Press (Machine) – 8 – 12 reps for 1 set.**
- **Lateral Raises (Machine) – 8 – 12 reps for 1 set.**
- **Biceps Curls (Machine) – 8 – 12 reps for 1 set.**
- **Triceps Extensions (Machine) – 8 – 12 reps for 1 set.**
- **Leg Press (Machine) – 8 – 12 reps for 1 set.**
- **Calves Press (Machine) – 8 – 12 reps for 1 set.**
- **Sit-Ups (Machine) – 8 – 12 reps for 1 set.**
- **Side-to-Sides (Machine) – 8 – 12 reps for 1 set.**
- **Back Extensions (Machine) – 8 – 12 reps for 1 set.**

Combined with aerobic training

- **30 – 60 minutes of walking/running/cycling/rowing/swimming/cross-training with an intensity of 47 – 52 % of VO2max. If you have an intensity over 52 % of VO2max, it doesn't matter that much, as long as you do your exercise. The intensity of 47 % - 52 % of VO2max is the peak rate of fat oxidation, and if you, for example, have an intensity of 75 % of VO2max, you will only have a decreased rate of fat oxidation but you will burn more calories.**

Notes on the workout

You will still perform 1 set per exercise. This time when you perform the exercises, you can try to find a weight that you can do for a minimum of 8 reps and a maximum of 12 reps. So, if you for example, took 10 kg (22.22 lbs) for 12 reps on the Bench Press at the last training session, then you can pick 12.5 kg (27.7 lbs) and try to perform at least 8 reps for 1 set.

On the core exercises (Sit-Ups, Side-to-Sides and Back Extensions), if you already could perform 12 reps on each of these exercises, then you can add weight 1 kg (2.22 lbs) to the exercises and try to perform 8 reps for 1 set.

On the aerobic exercise, if you, for example, performed 30 minutes of walking with a speed of 4 km/h (2.5 mph) at the last training session, then you can try to perform 32 minutes of walking of 4 km/h (2.5 mph).

Thursday

On this day, you will only perform aerobic training. For example, you can walk for 30 – 60 minutes, you can run for 30 – 60 minutes or spinning for 30 – 60 minutes in whatever pace you want, but try to hit at least 47 % - 52 % of your VO2max. If you, for example, walked for 30 minutes at the last training session, then you can try to cycle for 30 minutes this time or you can try to walk for 32 minutes.

Friday

- **Bench Press (Machine) – 8 – 12 reps for 1 set.**
- **Lat Pull Downs (Machine) – 8 – 12 reps for 1 set.**
- **Shoulder Press (Machine) – 8 – 12 reps for 1 set.**
- **Lateral Raises (Machine) – 8 – 12 reps for 1 set.**
- **Biceps Curls (Machine) – 8 – 12 reps for 1 set.**
- **Triceps Extensions (Machine) – 8 – 12 reps for 1 set.**
- **Leg Press (Machine) – 8 – 12 reps for 1 set.**
- **Calves Press (Machine) – 8 – 12 reps for 1 set.**
- **Sit-Ups (Machine) – 8 – 12 reps for 1 set.**
- **Side-to-Sides (Machine) – 8 – 12 reps for 1 set.**
- **Back Extensions (Machine) – 8 – 12 reps for 1 set.**

Combined with aerobic training

- **30 - 60 minutes of walking/running/cycling/rowing/swimming/cross-training with an intensity of 47 % – 52 % of**

VO2max. If you have an intensity over 52 % of VO2max, it doesn't matter that much, as long as you do your exercise. The intensity of 47 % - 52 % of VO2max is the peak rate of fat oxidation, and if you, for example, have an intensity of 75 % of VO2max, you will only have a decreased rate of fat oxidation but you will burn more calories.

Notes on the workout

I think you start to see the pattern of my workout plan. ALWAYS TRY TO PROGRESS! If you for example did 9 reps with the weight of 10 kg (22.22 lbs) on the bench press last training session, then you will try to perform 10 reps with the same weight. Even on the aerobic exercises, if you, for example, performed 32 minutes of walking with the speed of 4 km/h (2.5 mph), then you can try to walk for 34 minutes with the same speed or you can start to progress on another aerobic exercise, for example, the spinning cycle. Start with 30 minutes with a speed

(Watts) that you can hold through the entire training session.

The weekend

At the weekends, there is no specific training that you will do. Instead, you will increase the everyday activities and reduce the sedentary. You can for example, play with your kids in the park (if you are a parent), you can go for a walk, you can, instead of driving to the supermarket, walk to the supermarket (if it isn't too far away of course), you can take the stairs instead of the elevator if you live in an apartment, you can take a bicycle ride and have picnic with some fruits and berries on the way. You can do whatever you want, as long as you are active in some way for at least 30 minutes.

The exercises for week 2
Monday, Wednesday, Friday

- **Bench Press (Machine) – 8 – 12 reps for 1 set.**
- **Lat Pull Downs (Machine) – 8 – 12 reps for 1 set.**

- **Shoulder Press (Machine) – 8 – 12 reps for 1 set.**
- **Lateral Raises (Machine) – 8 – 12 reps for 1 set.**
- **Biceps Curls (Machine) – 8 – 12 reps for 1 set.**
- **Triceps Extensions (Machine) – 8 – 12 reps for 1 set.**
- **Leg Press (Machine) – 8 – 12 reps for 1 set.**
- **Calves Press (Machine) – 8 – 12 reps for 1 set.**
- **Sit-Ups (Machine) – 8 – 12 reps for 1 set.**
- **Side-to-Sides (Machine) – 8 – 12 reps for 1 set.**
- **Back Extensions (Machine) – 8 – 12 reps for 1 set.**

Combined with aerobic training

- **30 - 60 minutes of walking/running/cycling/rowing/swimming/cross-training with an intensity of 47 – 52 % of VO2max. If you have an intensity over 52 % of VO2max, it doesn't matter that much, as long as you do your exercise. The intensity of 47 % - 52 % of VO2max is the peak rate of fat**

**oxidation, and if you, for example, have an
intensity of 75 % of VO2max, you will only
have a decreased rate of fat oxidation but you
will burn more calories.**

Notes on the workout

This is your second week of training. You may have
some soreness from last week's training and that is
normal in the beginning. But the risk of injury increases
when we have soreness, therefore, we will still perform 1
set per exercise.

You will have the weights that you lifted with last Friday
and continue to progress on the exercises. So, if you did 9
reps for 1 set on the Shoulder Press last Friday, this time
you will try to perform 10 reps for 1 set. If you only can
perform 9 reps for one set, this means that you will try to
perform 10 reps for 1 set on Wednesday instead. You will
never increase the weight until you can perform 12 reps
for 1 set with proper form.

On the aerobic exercise, you will always increase the speed or the distance or switch exercise and increase the speed or the distance.

Tuesday and Thursday

On this day, you will only perform aerobic training. For example, you can walk for 30 – 60 minutes, you can run for 30 – 60 minutes or spinning for 30 – 60 minutes in whatever pace you want, but try to hit at least 47 % - 52 % of your VO2max. If you, for example, walked for 30 minutes at the last training session, then you can try to cycle for 30 minutes this time or you can try to walk for 32 minutes.

The weekend

At the weekends, there is no specific training that you will do. Instead, you will increase the everyday activities and reduce the sedentary. You can for example, play with your kids in the park (if you are a parent), you can go for a walk, you can, instead of driving to the supermarket, walk to the supermarket (if it isn't too far away of course), you can take the stairs instead of the elevator if you live in an apartment, you can take a bicycle ride and have picnic with some fruits and berries on the way. You can do whatever you want, as long as you are active in some way for at least 30 minutes.

Week 3 and until you have reached your goal body weight and/or goal body fat percentage

Monday, Wednesday, Friday

- **Bench Press (Machine) – 8 – 12 reps for 1 set.**
- **Lat Pull Downs (Machine) – 8 – 12 reps for 1 set.**
- **Shoulder Press (Machine) – 8 – 12 reps for 1 set.**
- **Lateral Raises (Machine) – 8 – 12 reps for 1 set.**
- **Biceps Curls (Machine) – 8 – 12 reps for 1 set.**
- **Triceps Extensions (Machine) – 8 – 12 reps for 1 set.**
- **Leg Press (Machine) – 8 – 12 reps for 1 set.**
- **Calves Press (Machine) – 8 – 12 reps for 1 set.**
- **Sit-Ups (Machine) – 8 – 12 reps for 1 set.**
- **Side-to-Sides (Machine) – 8 – 12 reps for 1 set.**

- **Back Extensions (Machine) – 8 – 12 reps for 1 set.**

Combined with aerobic training

- **30 - 60 minutes of walking/running/cycling/rowing/swimming/cross-training with an intensity of 47 – 52 % of VO2max. If you have an intensity over 52 % of VO2max, it doesn't matter that much, as long as you do your exercise. The intensity of 47 % - 52 % of VO2max is the peak rate of fat oxidation, and if you, for example, have an intensity of 75 % of VO2max, you will only have a decreased rate of fat oxidation but you will burn more calories.**

Notes on the workout

Now, you have become very comfortable with the exercises but you will still perform 8 – 12 reps with 1 set on the resistance exercises three days per week. You will only increase the workloads when you can perform 12 reps for 1 set with a proper form. The workloads will be increased with 2.22 lbs (1 kg) for each workout except for the leg press that will be increased with 5 lbs (2.25 kg). So, the method here is to always increase the reps until you can perform 12 reps with a proper form and then increase the weight until you can perform 12 reps again with the new weight.

For the aerobic exercises, you will always try to progress, either on the speed for a specific distance, maybe you want to run faster on 5K (5 kilometer – 3.1 miles) then you will increase the speed for every training session. Maybe you want to swim for a longer distance, then you don't need to increase the speed just try to reach the distance you want, and increase the speed from there. This principle applies to all endurance exercises. **"INCREASE THE SPEED FOR A GIVEN DISTANCE OR INCREASE THE DISTANCE WITHOUT INCREASING THE SPEED".**

Tuesday and Thursday

On this day, you will only perform aerobic training. For example, you can walk for 30 – 60 minutes, you can run for 30 – 60 minutes or spinning for 30 – 60 minutes in whatever pace you want, but try to hit at least 47 % - 52 % of your VO2max. If you, for example, walked for 30 minutes at the last training session, then you can try to cycle for 30 minutes this time or you can try to walk for 32 minutes. On these two days, you will always work with the aerobic endurance exercises, just to reduce the sedentary, and accordingly to the research above, aerobic exercises alone result in a greater weight loss than resistance training alone. I love walks and runs on these days, just being able to walk for 60 minutes and listen to a podcast or an audio book or just some music feels like freedom for many people. The walks and runs on these days aren't just beneficial for weight loss and fat burning, they are also a perfect time for learning, especially if you listen to audio books or a documentary about any topic you find interesting, because the brain memorizes more when you are working out.

The weekend

At the weekends, there is no specific training that you will do. Instead, you will increase the everyday activities and reduce the sedentary. You can, for example, play with your kids in the park (if you are a parent), you can go for a walk, you can, instead of driving to the supermarket, walk to the supermarket (if it isn't too far away of course), you can take the stairs instead of the elevator if you live in an apartment, you can take a bicycle ride and have picnic with some fruits and berries on the way. You can do whatever you want, as long as you are active in some way for at least 30 minutes.

Summary of the training program

You will perform 8 – 12 reps for 1 set on each exercise until you have reached your goal body weight or goal body fat percentage. You will **combine the resistance training with aerobic endurance exercises** and increase either the speed for a given distance or increase the distance without increasing the speed for all aerobic endurance exercises. **You will walk/run/swim/ride**

bicycle every Tuesday and Thursday through the entire program. **On the weekends**, you will increase the activity by having fun, for example, hike, climb mountains, go for shopping, ride the bicycles to a lake and have picnic with some fruits, swim, clean the house, go on a training pass that you enjoy (for example, yoga or a whole new training pass that you have never heard of before) etc.

Chapter 18

The training program (aerobic endurance exercise)

The training program that you just read above is the training program we will aim for and progress at. But, many of you don't want to exercise at the gym in the beginning and some of you can't do resistance training in the beginning because of your body weight. So, for you, I will create a separate training program that only includes aerobic endurance exercise. The goal with this program, is that you will reduce your body weight and body fat percentage to be able to follow the original training program. I can't tell you when you can start with the original training program, you must feel for yourself, and when you have the confidence to perform resistance training combined with aerobic endurance exercise, then you can start the original training program. But right now, we will only focus on aerobic endurance exercise and reducing the calorie intake so that you reduce body weight and body fat percentage in some way.

The types of aerobic endurance exercise you will use in this program are mainly walking, running (if you can), cycling, rowing, swimming, cross-training etc.
You will start very slowly just because we want to reduce the risk of injuries.

During this entire program, you will perform 30 – 60 minutes of walking/running/cycling/rowing/swimming/cross-training with an intensity of 47 % and 52 % of VO2max. If you have an intensity over 52 % of VO2max, it doesn't matter that much, as long as you do your exercise. The intensity of 47 % - 52 % of VO2max is the peak rate of fat oxidation, and if you, for example, have an intensity of 75 % of VO2max, you will only have a decreased rate of fat oxidation but you will burn more calories.

For the aerobic exercises, you will always try to progress, either on the speed for a specific distance, maybe you want to run faster on 5K (5 kilometer – 3.1 miles) then you will increase the speed for every training session. Maybe you want to swim for a longer distance, then you don't need to increase the speed just try to reach the distance you want, and increase the speed from there. This principle applies to all endurance exercises. **"INCREASE THE SPEED FOR A GIVEN DISTANCE OR INCREASE THE DISTANCE WITHOUT INCREASING THE SPEED".**

You will increase the speed for a given distance or increase the distance without increasing the speed three days per week, for example, on Monday, Wednesday and Friday. These days are the workout days. On the other four days of the week, you will just try to be as active as possible, but I would recommend to walk/run/swim/ride on the bicycle for at least 30 minutes just to reduce the sedentary.

You will perform this training program combined with a reduced calorie intake and with healthy food choices that you probably have reed in this book already.

This training program looks like this:

Monday – Workout day, perform 30 – 60 minutes of aerobic endurance exercise. You will increase the speed for a given distance or increase the distance without increasing the speed.

Tuesday – Be active for at least 30 minutes just by walking/running/swimming/cycling.

Wednesday - Workout day, perform 30 – 60 minutes of aerobic endurance exercises. You will increase the speed for a given distance or increase the distance without increasing the speed.

Thursday – Be active for at least 30 minutes just by walking/running/swimming/cycling.

Friday - Workout day, perform 30 – 60 minutes of aerobic endurance exercises. You will increase the speed for a given distance or increase the distance without increasing the speed.

Saturday - Be active for at least 30 minutes just by walking/running/swimming/cycling.

Sunday - Be active for at least 30 minutes just by walking/running/swimming/cycling.

Chapter 19

The program without the training part

Some of you people out there has a very heavy body weight and just because of that you won't be able to perform resistance training and aerobic endurance training right now because the risk of injuries is too high, but you will be able to perform those types of training programs when you have lost body weight. Some of you people might even have a hard time to move and your knees hurt when you move. Therefore, this training program is for you right now, but you will progress to the other programs when you have the confidence to do so and when you feel no pain in your knees.

So, this program is all about one thing, reducing the calorie intake and start to consume healthy foods to reduce the body weight and body fat percentage. You can find what healthy foods you will consume in this book during chapter 14 - good food selections based on NNR 2012. You will also find how many calories you must consume to lose body weight in the chapter below – how to calculate your maintenance level.

Chapter 20

How to calculate your maintenance level

When you consume as many calories as your body expends in a day is your maintenance level. The maintenance level can be calculated in some different ways, but I am going to use one equation and one easier way to calculate it. The first way is through an equation called Mifflin-St Jeor Equation which gives you a result based on your basal metabolic rate which is the calories you burn per day by just sitting at home. It is the calories you burn from just your cells' work (189).

The equation looks like this:

For men: Basal metabolic rate = 10 x weight (kg) + 6.25 x height (cm) – 5 x age (years) + 5
For women: Basal metabolic rate = 10 x weight (kg) + 6.25 x height (cm) – 5 x age (years) – 161 (189).

For example, if you weight 140 kg, is 180 cm and is 32 years old, then you follow the equation like this.

First, you multiply 10 with your body weight in kg (10 x 140 = 1400). Then you multiply 6.25 with your height in cm (6.25 x 180 = 1125). Then you multiply 5 with your age in years (5 x 32 = 160). Now, you have three different numbers and from now on, you will just put the numbers in the equation just like this: 1400 + 1125 – 160 + 5 = 2370 calories at rest if you are a man. If you are a woman, you do the same thing, but at the end of the equation you reduce with 161, just like this: 1400 + 1125 – 160 – 161 = 2204 calories at rest.

This is the calories you burn at rest. Now, many people don't just sit at home and do nothing all day in and all day out. Many people are walking to the work, take the bicycle to the gym, workout at the gym, go for a run, clean the house, go for shopping, etc. In this program, you will be active by working out at the gym three times per week and going for walks/runs two to four days per week. Therefore, we need a higher calorie intake than what the Mifflin-St Jeor equation shows us.

You can multiply the calories you burn at rest with 1.55 to get a number of calories that you burn from being active 5 – 7 days per week. So, if you are a man, in the example above, you multiply 2370 with 1.55 (2370 x 1.55 = 3673 calories) and if you are a woman, in the example above, you multiply 2204 with 1.55 (2204 x 1.55 = 3416 calories). If you consume this number of calories per day when you are active during the days by following the program, you will maintain your body weight. But, the goal of this program isn't to maintain our body weight until we have reached the body weight and body fat percentage we want; therefore, we need to burn fat and lose body weight. In this book, I mentioned that losing 1 lbs (0.45 kg) per week, you must lower your calorie intake with 500 calories. So, if you are burning 3673 calories per day, you will lower this intake with 500 calories, and it leaves you with 3173 calories per day, and if you are burning 3416 calories per day, you will lower this intake with 500 calories, and it leaves you with 2916 calories per day.

This is the first example of calculating your maintenance level. But remember, each week, you will lose body weight, and therefore, you will burn less calories than you did the last week, and this means that you must consume less calories to lose body weight. A good tip, is to do this equation again for your new body weight.

The second example is way easier than this example. The second example, is that you buy a Fitbit and type in your bodyweight, height and activity level, and the Fitbit calculates how many calories you must burn per day to reach your goal body weight. You can also do this on MyFitnessPal. This is an easier way to calculate your maintenance level, but if you are like me, you like challenges.

When you are following these calorie intakes, either from the equation or Fitbit/MyFitnessPal, if you gain body weight with the calculated calories, you can lower the calorie intake with 10 % or if you are losing weight too quickly (2 – 3 lbs (0.9 – 1.35 kg) per week), you can increase the calorie intake with 10 %. So, if you gain body weight, you multiply your current calorie intake with 0.90, so, for example, if you gain body weight with a calorie intake of 3173 calories, you multiply this number with 0.90 (3173 x 0.90 = 2856 calories), or if you gain body weight with a calorie intake of 2916 calories, you multiply this number with 0.90 (2916 x 0.90 = 2624 calories). If you, on the other hand, lose body weight too quickly, you can increase your current calorie intake with 10 %. So, if you lose body weight too quickly, you divide your current calorie intake with 0.90, so, for example, if you lose body weight too quickly with a calorie intake of 3173 calories, you divide this number with 0.90 (3173 / 0.90 = 3526 calories), or if you lose body weight too quickly with a calorie intake of 2916 calories, you divide this number with 0.90 (2916 / 0.90 = 3240 calories).

You will always weight yourself every morning at the same time to know if you have gained body weight, lost body weight or maintained body weight. But, the most important time to weight yourself is every Monday or Sunday at the same time which will show you if you have gained, lost or maintained your body weight during the week.

Chapter 21

Summary of the book – how to follow the structure

1. Fast 16 – 20 hours per day every day. Consume food 8 – 4 hours per day. Consume 1 – 3 meals per day depending on how much you can consume in one sitting.

2. Be in caloric deficit until you have reached your goal body weight, and then increase the calories so you are in maintenance.

3. Obesity is treated by a lower calorie intake than the body expends in a day.

4. Health benefits of intermittent fasting: Glucose- and lipid metabolism decreases, lipolysis and fat oxidation increases and blood sugar levels

decrease, lipolysis increase due to lowered concentration of plasma insulin, higher concentration of growth hormone and increased activity of sympathetic nervous system, concentrations of plasma fatty acids increase, level of plasma glycerol increases, decrease of glucose oxidation, increased energy expenditure due to increased concentrations of noradrenaline, increased beta hydroxybutyrate, plasma fatty acids, decrease of the levels of triglycerides and respiratory quotient, you can live longer, increased insulin sensitivity, increased glucose tolerance, increased fat mass loss combined with resistance training, increased fat free mass combined with resistance training, reduced levels of testosterone and IGF-1, improved HOMA-IR, increased adiponectin, decreased leptin, decreased levels of triglycerides, decreased T3, decreased TNF-alpha, decreased levels of IL-1 Beta, increased alertness/excitement, more focused and driven, increased mental acuity, improved physical performance.

5. Minimizing the loss of fat free mass may be achieved through bigger meals with more calories in the evenings.

6. 22 – 29 % protein of the energy intake results in less loss of fat free mass than 12 – 20 % protein of the energy intake. It doesn't matter when you consume the protein during the day, as long as you consume the protein.

7. Do not consume food after 8 PM because it is greater opportunities to develop increased BMI, obesity and decreased insulin sensitivity.

8. LCHF is not good for the health, it will increase the risk of cardiovascular disease.

9. Eat SMART – Larger share of vegetables, Less space for empty calories, Increase in organic growth, Proper meat and vegetable selection, Transport low.

10. According to NNR 2012, all individuals should: increase the intake of fish and seafood, fruits and berries, nuts and seeds and vegetables and pulses. Exchange butter and butter based spreads to vegetable oils and vegetable oil based fat spreads,

exchange high-fat dairy to low-fat dairy, and exchange refined cereals to wholegrain cereals. Limit the intake of salt, processed meat, red meat, alcohol and beverages and foods with added sugar.

11. An unbalanced diet should not be complemented with supplements that contain vitamins and minerals, instead the unbalanced diet should become balanced by increase the intake of the lacking vitamins.

12. A low energy intake is considered as 1552 calories – 1910 calories and a very low energy intake is considered as a calorie intake below 1552 calories, these intakes increase the risk of not consuming all micronutrients, and therefore, intakes below 1552 calories are recommended to be complemented with a multivitamin/mineral tablet for reaching the requirements of all the micronutrients.

13. It is very important to drink enough of water during the day.

14. "Physical activity includes all body movements of the skeletal muscle which results in increased energy turnover over the rest. Physical activity thus includes all body movements regardless of purpose or context".

15. Physical activity helps to reduce the risk of the development of cardiovascular diseases, helps to improve cognition, reduce depression, has a positive correlation with the body weight, improve fitness, increase muscular strength, increase lifespan, and preventing diabetes type 2.

16. More than 150 minutes of moderate physical activity per week helps to prevent weight gain and promote weight loss.

17. Physical activity also helps to counteract the negative consequences of obesity by reducing abdominal fat, increasing insulin sensitivity, changing lipids, reducing blood pressure, increasing rate of mobilization of fatty tissues, reducing subcutaneous fat, increasing metabolism and fat oxidation and increasing lipolysis activity in muscles, reduce the risk of colon cancer and

breast cancer, strengthen your bones and muscles and prevent older people to fall.

18. Start off very slowly with moderate physical activity if you are new to it, because the risk of heart attacks can increase when you perform an activity very intense that you aren't used to. It is better to gradually increase the activity level to avoid injuries. It is very important to have a dialogue with your doctor if you have diabetes, arthritis or heart disease before you start the training program and diet program. But it is important that you avoid being inactive.

19. Physical inactivity with the definition "Physical inactivity includes all activities that do not lead to an energy consumption over the one that is at rest. All activities corresponding to 1.0 – 1.5 MET". Physical inactivity can lead to harmful symptoms in the body.

20. Resistance training leads to some endocrine adjustments like increased testosterone, growth hormone, cortisol, norepinephrine, adrenaline, IGF-1 and insulin.

21. Benefits with strength training machines: good muscle building, easier for beginners, steered movement, good rehabilitation and exercises training, working with thoughtful muscle, small injury risk and a great way to know the muscles.

22. Disadvantages with strength training machines: they are rarely so well-designed that it suits all individuals, increase in strength is not transferred to sport, small/no stimulus on the stabilization muscles, slow motion, explosive strength training is difficult to implement.

23. Benefits with free weights: develops good mobility, good training for active athletes, infinite variation of each type of exercise, good muscle building, effective in both concentric and eccentric phase, develops speed and explosiveness, great stimulation on stabilization muscles, allows multi-level movements and is versatile.

24. Disadvantages with free weights: sometimes additional assistants are needed, may give lower transmission power in relation to sports

momentum, main resistance in the vertical plane, in case of wrong load the damage risk increases.

25. The recommendations of physical activity according to NNR 2012 are for adults: 150 minutes of moderate intensity exercise or 75 minutes of high intensity per week. For children and adolescents: 60 minutes' moderate to very stressful physical activity per day. Everyone is recommended to reduce the sedentary.

26. Drink water before, during and after the exercise. You should drink 150 % or more water of the weight loss if you have exercised for a long time, like running for 90 minutes.

27. Sleep for 7 – 9 hours per day if you are between 18 and 64 years old.

28. Choose BMI or DEXA scan for measuring your body composition.

29. It is very important to consume enough of micronutrients and macronutrients to lose weight in a healthy way.

30. The recommended intake of carbohydrates is 45 – 60 % of the total energy intake. The

recommended intake of added sugar should be kept below 10 % of the total energy intake. The recommended intake of dietary fibers should be 25 g or more per day for women and 35 g or more per day for men.

31. The recommended intake of protein is 10 – 20 % of the total energy intake which corresponds to about 0.8 – 1.5 g protein / kg body weight per day for adults. Less lean body mass is lost when the protein intake is between 13 – 20 % of the total energy intake.

32. The recommended intake of total fat is 25 – 40 % of the total energy intake. The recommended intake of monounsaturated fat is 10 – 20 % of the total energy intake. The recommended intake of polyunsaturated fat is 5 – 10 % of the total energy intake. The recommended intake of n-3 (omega-3) fat should be kept equal or over 1 % of the total energy intake. The recommended intake of saturated fat should be kept below 10 % of the total energy intake. The recommended intake of

trans-fatty acids should be as low as possible of the total energy intake.

33. It takes about 3500 calories to lose 1 lbs (0.45 kg) of fat which means that you must lower your calories with 500 – 1000 calories under your maintenance to lose 1 lbs (0.45 kg) of fat per week.

34. MyFitnessPal and Fitbit are great options for tracking your calories that you consume from the food and that you burn through physical activity.

35. You will consume vegetables and root vegetables, legumes, fruits and berries, nuts and seeds, cereal products, whole grain products, fiber-rich foods, more monounsaturated- and polyunsaturated fatty acids than saturated- and trans fatty acids, lean milk products, eggs, fish and seafood, lower intakes of red meat and processed meat products, lower intake of salt and salty foods, lower intake of energy-rich- and sugar-sourced foods, lower intake of alcoholic beverages and a higher intake of water because all these food sources result in lower risk of chronic disease.

36. Green tea, black tea and coffee have many health benefits and they are perfect to consume when you are fasting. You should consume the drinks before your workout which will give you more energy during the workout. You will also consume the drinks before your meal/meals which will result in that your appetite suppresses and you will consume fewer calories than you would do without tea or coffee before the meal/meals. Do not consume the drinks too late in the evenings, because some people have a harder time to sleep due to the caffeine, and the sleep is very important for your weight loss journey.

37. You will perform 8 – 12 reps for 1 set on each exercise until you have reached your goal body weight or goal body fat percentage. You will **combine the resistance training with aerobic endurance exercises** and increase either the speed for a given distance or increase the distance without increasing the speed for all aerobic endurance exercises. **You will walk/run/swim/ride bicycle every Tuesday and**

Thursday through the entire program. **On the weekends**, you will increase the activity by having fun, for example, hike, climb mountains, go for shopping, ride the bicycles to a lake and have picnic with some fruits, swim, clean the house, go on a training pass that you enjoy (for example, yoga or a whole new training pass that you have never heard of before) etc.

38. If you can't or won't be able to perform resistance training combined with aerobic endurance training, then you can follow the program 'the training program (aerobic endurance exercise)' which will only focus on aerobic endurance exercises and reducing the calorie intake and eating healthy foods for body weight loss and body fat percentage reduction. You will do some type of endurance exercise every day for at least 30 minutes a day. It can be walking, running, cycling, swimming etc. Follow this program until you have the confidence and can be able to perform resistance training combined with aerobic endurance training.

39. Some of you won't be able to perform any type of exercise (resistance training and/or endurance training) when you buy this program because you might have a very heavy body weight right now or you feel pain in your knees when you move, and for you, I have decided that you will only focus on reducing the calorie intake, consuming healthy foods to reduce the body weight and the body fat percentage.

40. Weight yourself every morning at the same time, or every Monday or Sunday at the same time to know if you have gained, lost or maintained body weight during the week.

Good Luck!

I believe in you and I always will!

Pontus Olsson

References

1. Moro T, Tinsley G, Bianco A, Marcolin G,
   Pacelli QF, Battaglia G, et al.
   Effects of eight weeks of time-
   restricted feeding (16/8)
   on basal metabolism, maximal strength, body com
   position, inflammation,
   and cardiovascular risk factors in resistance-
   trained males. J Transl Med. 2016 Oct
   13;14(1):290.

2. Tinsley GM, La Bounty PM.
   Effects of intermittent fasting on body compositio
   n and clinical health markers in humans. Nutr
   Rev. 2015 Oct;73(10):661-74.

3. Gotthardt JD, Bello NT.
   Meal pattern alterations associated with intermitte
   nt fasting for weight loss are normalized after
   high-fat diet re-feeding. Physiol Behav. 2017 May
   15;174:49-56.

4. Wolke E. Ätstörningar [PowerPoint presentation on the Internet]. Kalmar: Linnéuniversitetet; 2016. [cited March 8 2017]. Available from: https://mymoodle.lnu.se/pluginfile.php/1389759/mod_resource/content/1/ABC%20-%20mottagningen%20Ätstörningar%20Eva%20Wolke.pdf.

5. 1177 Vårdguiden. Bulimi [Internet]. Stockholm: 1177 Vårdguiden; 2017 [updated date 2017-02-06; cited 2017 March 8]. Available from: https://www.1177.se/Kronoberg/Fakta-och-rad/Sjukdomar/Bulimi/.

6. Andersson H. Energi och metabolism [PowerPoint presentation on the Internet]. Kalmar: Linnéuniversitetet; 2016. [cited March 14 2017]. Available from: https://mymoodle.lnu.se/pluginfile.php/1318211/mod_resource/content/3/Lectures/Energibalans.pdf.

7. Hatting M, Rines AK, Luo C, Tabata M, Sharabi K, Hall JA, et al.

317

Adipose Tissue CLK2 Promotes Energy Expendit
ure during High-Fat Diet Intermittent Fasting.
Cell Metab. 2017 Feb 7;25(2):428-437.

8. Shi H, Akunuru S, Bierman JC, Hodge KM,
   Mitchell MC, Foster MT, et al. Diet-induced
   obese mice are leptin insufficient after weight
   reduction. Obesity (Silver Spring). 2009
   Sep;17(9):1702-9.

9. Chung H, Chou W, Sears DD, Patterson RE,
   Webster NJ, Ellies LG. Time-
   restricted feeding improves insulin resistance and
   hepatic steatosis in
   a mouse model of postmenopausal obesity.
   Metabolism. 2016 Dec;65(12):1743-1754.

10. Nseir W, Hellou E, Assy N. Role of diet and
    lifestyle changes in nonalcoholic fatty liver
    disease. World J Gastroenterol. 2014 Jul
    28;20(28):9338-44.

11. Mattson MP, Longo VD, Harvie M. Impact of
    intermittent fasting on health and disease
    processes. Ageing Res Rev. 2017 Oct;39:46-58.

12. Napolitano MA, Hayes S. Behavioral and psychological factors associated w ith 12-month weight change in a physical activity trial. J Obes. 2011;2011:515803.

13. Keim NL, Van Loan MD, Horn WF, Barbieri TF, Mayclin PL. Weight loss is greater with consumption of large morning meals and fat-free mass is preservedwith large evening meals in women on a controlled weight reduction regimen. J Nutr. 1997 Jan;127(1):75-82.

14. Harvey-Berino J. Calorie restriction is more effective for obesity treatment than dietary fat restriction. Ann Behav Med. 1999 Spring;21(1):35-9.

15. Phelan S, Wyatt H, Nassery S, Dibello J, Fava JL, Hill JO, et al. Three-year weight change in successful weight losers who lost weight on a low-carbohydrate diet. Obesity (Silver Spring). 2007 Oct;15(10):2470-7.

16. Adechian S, Rémond D, Gaudichon C, Dardevet D, Mosoni L. The nature of the ingested protein

has no effect on lean body mass during energy restriction in overweight rats. Obesity (Silver Spring). 2011 Jun;19(6):1137-44.

17. Westerterp-Plantenga MS. The significance of protein in food intake and body weight regulation. Curr Opin Clin Nutr Metab Care. 2003 Nov;6(6):635-8.

18. Examine. Protein and Intentional Weight Loss [Internet]. Toronto: Examine; 2012 [updated date 2012-09-01; 2017 April 5]. Available from: https://examine.com/nutrition/how-does-protein-affect-weight-loss/.

19. Garaulet M, Gómez-Abellán P, Alburquerque-Béjar JJ, Lee Y-C, Ordovás JM, Scheer FAJL. Timing of food intake predicts weight loss effectiveness. Int J Obes (Lond). 2013 Apr;37(4):604-611.

20. Paulún F. 50 genvägar till fettförbränning. Falun: ScandBook AB; 2014. P. 23

21. Paulún F. 50 genvägar till fettförbränning. Falun: ScandBook AB; 2014. P. 24

22. Witthöft C. Livsmedelskvalitet [PowerPoint presentation on the Internet]. Kalmar: Linnéuniversitetet; 2015. [cited April 8 2017]. Available from: https://mymoodle.lnu.se/pluginfile.php/1153071/mod_resource/content/1/livsmedelskvalitet20151029%206.pdf.

23. Nordic Nutrition Recommendations 2012: Integrating nutrition and physical activity. 5th ed. Copenhagen: Nordic Nutrition Recommendations 2012; 2014 [cited 2017-11-05]. 627 p (Nord). Available from: http://www.norden.org/en/theme/former-themes/themes-2016/nordic-nutrition-recommendation/nordic-nutrition-recommendations-2012 p. 23.

24. Nordic Nutrition Recommendations 2012: Integrating nutrition and physical activity. 5th ed. Copenhagen: Nordic Nutrition Recommendations 2012; 2014 [cited 2017-11-05]. 627 p (Nord). Available from: http://www.norden.org/en/theme/former-

themes/themes-2016/nordic-nutrition-
recommendation/nordic-nutrition-
recommendations-2012 p. 32.

25. Nordic Nutrition Recommendations 2012:
Integrating nutrition and physical activity. 5th ed.
Copenhagen: Nordic Nutrition Recommendations
2012; 2014 [cited 2017-11-05]. 627 p (Nord).
Available from:
http://www.norden.org/en/theme/former-
themes/themes-2016/nordic-nutrition-
recommendation/nordic-nutrition-
recommendations-2012 p. 33.

26. Nordic Nutrition Recommendations 2012:
Integrating nutrition and physical activity. 5th ed.
Copenhagen: Nordic Nutrition Recommendations
2012; 2014 [cited 2017-11-05]. 627 p (Nord).
Available from:
http://www.norden.org/en/theme/former-
themes/themes-2016/nordic-nutrition-
recommendation/nordic-nutrition-
recommendations-2012 p. 158.

27. Bergman P. Vad är fysisk aktivitet? [PowerPoint presentation on the Internet]. Kalmar: Linnéuniversitetet; 2016. [cited October 4 2017]. Available from: https://connect.sunet.se/p9nqjezuyo0/?launcher=false&fcsContent=true&pbMode=normal.

28. Ahlgren M. Idrottsnutrition [PowerPoint presentation on the Internet]. Kalmar: Linnéuniversitetet; 2016. [cited October 9 2017]. Available from: https://mymoodle.lnu.se/pluginfile.php/1425206/mod_resource/content/1/Handouts%20Idrottsnutrition.pdf.

29. Centers for Disease Control and Prevention. Physical activity and health [Internet]. USA: Centers for Disease Control and Prevention; 2015 [updated date 2015-06-04; cited 2017 October 8 2017]. Available from: https://www.cdc.gov/physicalactivity/basics/pa-health/index.htm.

30. Nordic Nutrition Recommendations 2012: Integrating nutrition and physical activity. 5th ed. Copenhagen: Nordic Nutrition Recommendations 2012; 2014 [cited 2017-10-06]. 627 p (Nord). Available from: http://www.norden.org/en/theme/former-themes/themes-2016/nordic-nutrition-recommendation/nordic-nutrition-recommendations-2012 p. 195.

31. Hirshkowitz M, Whiton K, Albert SM, Alessi C, Bruni O, DonCarlos L, et al. National sleep foundation's sleep time duration recommendations: methodology and results summary. Sleep Health. 2015 Mar;1(1):40-43.

32. Persson AA. GI-kanalen [PowerPoint presentation on the Internet]. Kalmar: Linnéuniversitetet; 2015. [cited September 19 2017]. Available from: https://mymoodle.lnu.se/mod/folder/view.php?id=829732.

33. Andersson H. Matspjälkningsprocessen [PowerPoint presentation on the Internet].

Kalmar: Linnéuniversitetet; 2016. [cited
September 20 2017]. Available from:
https://mymoodle.lnu.se/pluginfile.php/1318193/
mod_resource/content/4/Lectures/Introduktion%2
0%2B%20matspjälkning.pdf.

34. Nordic Nutrition Recommendations 2012:
    Integrating nutrition and physical activity. 5th ed.
    Copenhagen: Nordic Nutrition Recommendations
    2012; 2014 [cited 2017-11-06]. 627 p (Nord).
    Available from:
    http://www.norden.org/en/theme/former-
    themes/themes-2016/nordic-nutrition-
    recommendation/nordic-nutrition-
    recommendations-2012 p. 24.

35. Nordic Nutrition Recommendations 2012:
    Integrating nutrition and physical activity. 5th ed.
    Copenhagen: Nordic Nutrition Recommendations
    2012; 2014 [cited 2017-11-09]. 627 p (Nord).
    Available from:
    http://www.norden.org/en/theme/former-
    themes/themes-2016/nordic-nutrition-

recommendation/nordic-nutrition-recommendations-2012 p. 515.

36. Nordic Nutrition Recommendations 2012: Integrating nutrition and physical activity. 5th ed. Copenhagen: Nordic Nutrition Recommendations 2012; 2014 [cited 2017-11-09]. 627 p (Nord). Available from: http://www.norden.org/en/theme/former-themes/themes-2016/nordic-nutrition-recommendation/nordic-nutrition-recommendations-2012 p. 516.

37. Nordic Nutrition Recommendations 2012: Integrating nutrition and physical activity. 5th ed. Copenhagen: Nordic Nutrition Recommendations 2012; 2014 [cited 2017-11-09]. 627 p (Nord). Available from: http://www.norden.org/en/theme/former-themes/themes-2016/nordic-nutrition-recommendation/nordic-nutrition-recommendations-2012 p. 517.

38. Nordic Nutrition Recommendations 2012: Integrating nutrition and physical activity. 5th ed.

Copenhagen: Nordic Nutrition Recommendations 2012; 2014 [cited 2017-11-09]. 627 p (Nord). Available from: http://www.norden.org/en/theme/former-themes/themes-2016/nordic-nutrition-recommendation/nordic-nutrition-recommendations-2012 p. 528.

39. Witthöft C. Bone Health [PowerPoint presentation on the Internet]. Kalmar: Linnéuniversitetet; 2016. [cited June 25 2017]. Available from: https://mymoodle.lnu.se/pluginfile.php/1385412/mod_resource/content/1/BenhälsaMineralämnen20160408.pdf.

40. Nordic Nutrition Recommendations 2012: Integrating nutrition and physical activity. 5th ed. Copenhagen: Nordic Nutrition Recommendations 2012; 2014 [cited 2017-11-09]. 627 p (Nord). Available from: http://www.norden.org/en/theme/former-themes/themes-2016/nordic-nutrition-

recommendation/nordic-nutrition-recommendations-2012 p. 475.

41. Nordic Nutrition Recommendations 2012: Integrating nutrition and physical activity. 5th ed. Copenhagen: Nordic Nutrition Recommendations 2012; 2014 [cited 2017-11-09]. 627 p (Nord). Available from: http://www.norden.org/en/theme/former-themes/themes-2016/nordic-nutrition-recommendation/nordic-nutrition-recommendations-2012 p. 476.

42. Nordic Nutrition Recommendations 2012: Integrating nutrition and physical activity. 5th ed. Copenhagen: Nordic Nutrition Recommendations 2012; 2014 [cited 2017-11-09]. 627 p (Nord). Available from: http://www.norden.org/en/theme/former-themes/themes-2016/nordic-nutrition-recommendation/nordic-nutrition-recommendations-2012 p. 477.

43. Nordic Nutrition Recommendations 2012: Integrating nutrition and physical activity. 5th ed.

Copenhagen: Nordic Nutrition Recommendations
2012; 2014 [cited 2017-11-10]. 627 p (Nord).
Available from:
http://www.norden.org/en/theme/former-
themes/themes-2016/nordic-nutrition-
recommendation/nordic-nutrition-
recommendations-2012 p. 535.

44. Nordic Nutrition Recommendations 2012:
Integrating nutrition and physical activity. 5th ed.
Copenhagen: Nordic Nutrition Recommendations
2012; 2014 [cited 2017-11-10]. 627 p (Nord).
Available from:
http://www.norden.org/en/theme/former-
themes/themes-2016/nordic-nutrition-
recommendation/nordic-nutrition-
recommendations-2012 p. 536.

45. Nordic Nutrition Recommendations 2012:
Integrating nutrition and physical activity. 5th ed.
Copenhagen: Nordic Nutrition Recommendations
2012; 2014 [cited 2017-11-10]. 627 p (Nord).
Available from:
http://www.norden.org/en/theme/former-

themes/themes-2016/nordic-nutrition-recommendation/nordic-nutrition-recommendations-2012 p. 539.

46. Nordic Nutrition Recommendations 2012: Integrating nutrition and physical activity. 5th ed. Copenhagen: Nordic Nutrition Recommendations 2012; 2014 [cited 2017-11-10]. 627 p (Nord). Available from: http://www.norden.org/en/theme/former-themes/themes-2016/nordic-nutrition-recommendation/nordic-nutrition-recommendations-2012 p. 540.

47. Nordic Nutrition Recommendations 2012: Integrating nutrition and physical activity. 5th ed. Copenhagen: Nordic Nutrition Recommendations 2012; 2014 [cited 2017-11-11]. 627 p (Nord). Available from: http://www.norden.org/en/theme/former-themes/themes-2016/nordic-nutrition-recommendation/nordic-nutrition-recommendations-2012 p. 501.

48. Nordic Nutrition Recommendations 2012:
Integrating nutrition and physical activity. 5th ed.
Copenhagen: Nordic Nutrition Recommendations
2012; 2014 [cited 2017-11-11]. 627 p (Nord).
Available from:
http://www.norden.org/en/theme/former-
themes/themes-2016/nordic-nutrition-
recommendation/nordic-nutrition-
recommendations-2012 p. 502.

49. Nordic Nutrition Recommendations 2012:
Integrating nutrition and physical activity. 5th ed.
Copenhagen: Nordic Nutrition Recommendations
2012; 2014 [cited 2017-11-11]. 627 p (Nord).
Available from:
http://www.norden.org/en/theme/former-
themes/themes-2016/nordic-nutrition-
recommendation/nordic-nutrition-
recommendations-2012 p. 503.

50. Nordic Nutrition Recommendations 2012:
Integrating nutrition and physical activity. 5th ed.
Copenhagen: Nordic Nutrition Recommendations
2012; 2014 [cited 2017-11-11]. 627 p (Nord).

Available from:

http://www.norden.org/en/theme/former-themes/themes-2016/nordic-nutrition-recommendation/nordic-nutrition-recommendations-2012 p. 509.

51. Nordic Nutrition Recommendations 2012: Integrating nutrition and physical activity. 5th ed. Copenhagen: Nordic Nutrition Recommendations 2012; 2014 [cited 2017-11-11]. 627 p (Nord). Available from:

http://www.norden.org/en/theme/former-themes/themes-2016/nordic-nutrition-recommendation/nordic-nutrition-recommendations-2012 p. 510.

52. Witthöft C. Trace elements [PowerPoint presentation on the Internet]. Kalmar: Linnéuniversitetet; 2016. [cited June 25 2017]. Available from:

https://mymoodle.lnu.se/pluginfile.php/1385415/mod_resource/content/1/Trace%20elements%202 0160408.pdf.

53. Nordic Nutrition Recommendations 2012: Integrating nutrition and physical activity. 5th ed. Copenhagen: Nordic Nutrition Recommendations 2012; 2014 [cited 2017-11-12]. 627 p (Nord). Available from: http://www.norden.org/en/theme/former-themes/themes-2016/nordic-nutrition-recommendation/nordic-nutrition-recommendations-2012 p. 545.

54. Nordic Nutrition Recommendations 2012: Integrating nutrition and physical activity. 5th ed. Copenhagen: Nordic Nutrition Recommendations 2012; 2014 [cited 2017-11-12]. 627 p (Nord). Available from: http://www.norden.org/en/theme/former-themes/themes-2016/nordic-nutrition-recommendation/nordic-nutrition-recommendations-2012 p. 547.

55. Nordic Nutrition Recommendations 2012: Integrating nutrition and physical activity. 5th ed. Copenhagen: Nordic Nutrition Recommendations 2012; 2014 [cited 2017-11-12]. 627 p (Nord).

Available from:

http://www.norden.org/en/theme/former-themes/themes-2016/nordic-nutrition-recommendation/nordic-nutrition-recommendations-2012 p. 559.

56. Nordic Nutrition Recommendations 2012: Integrating nutrition and physical activity. 5th ed. Copenhagen: Nordic Nutrition Recommendations 2012; 2014 [cited 2017-11-12]. 627 p (Nord). Available from: http://www.norden.org/en/theme/former-themes/themes-2016/nordic-nutrition-recommendation/nordic-nutrition-recommendations-2012 p. 543.

57. Nordic Nutrition Recommendations 2012: Integrating nutrition and physical activity. 5th ed. Copenhagen: Nordic Nutrition Recommendations 2012; 2014 [cited 2017-11-12]. 627 p (Nord). Available from: http://www.norden.org/en/theme/former-themes/themes-2016/nordic-nutrition-

recommendation/nordic-nutrition-recommendations-2012 p. 573.

58. Nordic Nutrition Recommendations 2012: Integrating nutrition and physical activity. 5th ed. Copenhagen: Nordic Nutrition Recommendations 2012; 2014 [cited 2017-11-12]. 627 p (Nord). Available from: http://www.norden.org/en/theme/former-themes/themes-2016/nordic-nutrition-recommendation/nordic-nutrition-recommendations-2012 p. 574.

59. Nordic Nutrition Recommendations 2012: Integrating nutrition and physical activity. 5th ed. Copenhagen: Nordic Nutrition Recommendations 2012; 2014 [cited 2017-11-12]. 627 p (Nord). Available from: http://www.norden.org/en/theme/former-themes/themes-2016/nordic-nutrition-recommendation/nordic-nutrition-recommendations-2012 p. 575.

60. Nordic Nutrition Recommendations 2012: Integrating nutrition and physical activity. 5th ed.

Copenhagen: Nordic Nutrition Recommendations 2012; 2014 [cited 2017-11-13]. 627 p (Nord). Available from: http://www.norden.org/en/theme/former-themes/themes-2016/nordic-nutrition-recommendation/nordic-nutrition-recommendations-2012 p. 583.

61. Nordic Nutrition Recommendations 2012: Integrating nutrition and physical activity. 5th ed. Copenhagen: Nordic Nutrition Recommendations 2012; 2014 [cited 2017-11-13]. 627 p (Nord). Available from: http://www.norden.org/en/theme/former-themes/themes-2016/nordic-nutrition-recommendation/nordic-nutrition-recommendations-2012 p. 584.

62. Nordic Nutrition Recommendations 2012: Integrating nutrition and physical activity. 5th ed. Copenhagen: Nordic Nutrition Recommendations 2012; 2014 [cited 2017-11-13]. 627 p (Nord). Available from: http://www.norden.org/en/theme/former-

themes/themes-2016/nordic-nutrition-recommendation/nordic-nutrition-recommendations-2012 p. 585.

63. Nordic Nutrition Recommendations 2012: Integrating nutrition and physical activity. 5th ed. Copenhagen: Nordic Nutrition Recommendations 2012; 2014 [cited 2017-11-13]. 627 p (Nord). Available from: http://www.norden.org/en/theme/former-themes/themes-2016/nordic-nutrition-recommendation/nordic-nutrition-recommendations-2012 p. 587.

64. Nordic Nutrition Recommendations 2012: Integrating nutrition and physical activity. 5th ed. Copenhagen: Nordic Nutrition Recommendations 2012; 2014 [cited 2017-11-13]. 627 p (Nord). Available from: http://www.norden.org/en/theme/former-themes/themes-2016/nordic-nutrition-recommendation/nordic-nutrition-recommendations-2012 p. 586.

65. Nordic Nutrition Recommendations 2012: Integrating nutrition and physical activity. 5th ed. Copenhagen: Nordic Nutrition Recommendations 2012; 2014 [cited 2017-11-13]. 627 p (Nord). Available from: http://www.norden.org/en/theme/former-themes/themes-2016/nordic-nutrition-recommendation/nordic-nutrition-recommendations-2012 p. 591.

66. Nordic Nutrition Recommendations 2012: Integrating nutrition and physical activity. 5th ed. Copenhagen: Nordic Nutrition Recommendations 2012; 2014 [cited 2017-11-13]. 627 p (Nord). Available from: http://www.norden.org/en/theme/former-themes/themes-2016/nordic-nutrition-recommendation/nordic-nutrition-recommendations-2012 p. 592.

67. Nordic Nutrition Recommendations 2012: Integrating nutrition and physical activity. 5th ed. Copenhagen: Nordic Nutrition Recommendations 2012; 2014 [cited 2017-11-13]. 627 p (Nord).

Available from:

http://www.norden.org/en/theme/former-themes/themes-2016/nordic-nutrition-recommendation/nordic-nutrition-recommendations-2012 p. 593.

68. Nordic Nutrition Recommendations 2012: Integrating nutrition and physical activity. 5th ed. Copenhagen: Nordic Nutrition Recommendations 2012; 2014 [cited 2017-11-13]. 627 p (Nord). Available from: http://www.norden.org/en/theme/former-themes/themes-2016/nordic-nutrition-recommendation/nordic-nutrition-recommendations-2012 p. 594.

69. Nordic Nutrition Recommendations 2012: Integrating nutrition and physical activity. 5th ed. Copenhagen: Nordic Nutrition Recommendations 2012; 2014 [cited 2017-11-13]. 627 p (Nord). Available from: http://www.norden.org/en/theme/former-themes/themes-2016/nordic-nutrition-

recommendation/nordic-nutrition-recommendations-2012 p. 597.

70. Nordic Nutrition Recommendations 2012: Integrating nutrition and physical activity. 5th ed. Copenhagen: Nordic Nutrition Recommendations 2012; 2014 [cited 2017-11-14]. 627 p (Nord). Available from: http://www.norden.org/en/theme/former-themes/themes-2016/nordic-nutrition-recommendation/nordic-nutrition-recommendations-2012 p. 601.

71. Nordic Nutrition Recommendations 2012: Integrating nutrition and physical activity. 5th ed. Copenhagen: Nordic Nutrition Recommendations 2012; 2014 [cited 2017-11-14]. 627 p (Nord). Available from: http://www.norden.org/en/theme/former-themes/themes-2016/nordic-nutrition-recommendation/nordic-nutrition-recommendations-2012 p. 602.

72. Nordic Nutrition Recommendations 2012: Integrating nutrition and physical activity. 5th ed.

Copenhagen: Nordic Nutrition Recommendations 2012; 2014 [cited 2017-11-14]. 627 p (Nord). Available from: http://www.norden.org/en/theme/former-themes/themes-2016/nordic-nutrition-recommendation/nordic-nutrition-recommendations-2012 p. 603.

73. Nordic Nutrition Recommendations 2012: Integrating nutrition and physical activity. 5th ed. Copenhagen: Nordic Nutrition Recommendations 2012; 2014 [cited 2017-11-14]. 627 p (Nord). Available from: http://www.norden.org/en/theme/former-themes/themes-2016/nordic-nutrition-recommendation/nordic-nutrition-recommendations-2012 p. 604.

74. Nordic Nutrition Recommendations 2012: Integrating nutrition and physical activity. 5th ed. Copenhagen: Nordic Nutrition Recommendations 2012; 2014 [cited 2017-11-14]. 627 p (Nord). Available from: http://www.norden.org/en/theme/former-

themes/themes-2016/nordic-nutrition-recommendation/nordic-nutrition-recommendations-2012 p. 605.

75. Nordic Nutrition Recommendations 2012: Integrating nutrition and physical activity. 5th ed. Copenhagen: Nordic Nutrition Recommendations 2012; 2014 [cited 2017-11-14]. 627 p (Nord). Available from: http://www.norden.org/en/theme/former-themes/themes-2016/nordic-nutrition-recommendation/nordic-nutrition-recommendations-2012 p. 607.

76. Nordic Nutrition Recommendations 2012: Integrating nutrition and physical activity. 5th ed. Copenhagen: Nordic Nutrition Recommendations 2012; 2014 [cited 2017-11-14]. 627 p (Nord). Available from: http://www.norden.org/en/theme/former-themes/themes-2016/nordic-nutrition-recommendation/nordic-nutrition-recommendations-2012 p. 608.

77. Nordic Nutrition Recommendations 2012: Integrating nutrition and physical activity. 5th ed. Copenhagen: Nordic Nutrition Recommendations 2012; 2014 [cited 2017-11-14]. 627 p (Nord). Available from: http://www.norden.org/en/theme/former-themes/themes-2016/nordic-nutrition-recommendation/nordic-nutrition-recommendations-2012 p. 610.

78. Nordic Nutrition Recommendations 2012: Integrating nutrition and physical activity. 5th ed. Copenhagen: Nordic Nutrition Recommendations 2012; 2014 [cited 2017-11-14]. 627 p (Nord). Available from: http://www.norden.org/en/theme/former-themes/themes-2016/nordic-nutrition-recommendation/nordic-nutrition-recommendations-2012 p. 609.

79. Nordic Nutrition Recommendations 2012: Integrating nutrition and physical activity. 5th ed. Copenhagen: Nordic Nutrition Recommendations 2012; 2014 [cited 2017-11-14]. 627 p (Nord).

Available from:

http://www.norden.org/en/theme/former-themes/themes-2016/nordic-nutrition-recommendation/nordic-nutrition-recommendations-2012 p. 613.

80. Nordic Nutrition Recommendations 2012: Integrating nutrition and physical activity. 5th ed. Copenhagen: Nordic Nutrition Recommendations 2012; 2014 [cited 2017-11-14]. 627 p (Nord). Available from:

http://www.norden.org/en/theme/former-themes/themes-2016/nordic-nutrition-recommendation/nordic-nutrition-recommendations-2012 p. 614.

81. Nordic Nutrition Recommendations 2012: Integrating nutrition and physical activity. 5th ed. Copenhagen: Nordic Nutrition Recommendations 2012; 2014 [cited 2017-11-14]. 627 p (Nord). Available from:

http://www.norden.org/en/theme/former-themes/themes-2016/nordic-nutrition-

recommendation/nordic-nutrition-
recommendations-2012 p. 615.

82. Nordic Nutrition Recommendations 2012:
Integrating nutrition and physical activity. 5th ed.
Copenhagen: Nordic Nutrition Recommendations
2012; 2014 [cited 2017-11-15]. 627 p (Nord).
Available from:
http://www.norden.org/en/theme/former-
themes/themes-2016/nordic-nutrition-
recommendation/nordic-nutrition-
recommendations-2012 p. 617.

83. Nordic Nutrition Recommendations 2012:
Integrating nutrition and physical activity. 5th ed.
Copenhagen: Nordic Nutrition Recommendations
2012; 2014 [cited 2017-11-15]. 627 p (Nord).
Available from:
http://www.norden.org/en/theme/former-
themes/themes-2016/nordic-nutrition-
recommendation/nordic-nutrition-
recommendations-2012 p. 618.

84. Nordic Nutrition Recommendations 2012:
Integrating nutrition and physical activity. 5th ed.

Copenhagen: Nordic Nutrition Recommendations 2012; 2014 [cited 2017-11-15]. 627 p (Nord). Available from: http://www.norden.org/en/theme/former-themes/themes-2016/nordic-nutrition-recommendation/nordic-nutrition-recommendations-2012 p. 619.

85. Nordic Nutrition Recommendations 2012: Integrating nutrition and physical activity. 5th ed. Copenhagen: Nordic Nutrition Recommendations 2012; 2014 [cited 2017-11-15]. 627 p (Nord). Available from: http://www.norden.org/en/theme/former-themes/themes-2016/nordic-nutrition-recommendation/nordic-nutrition-recommendations-2012 p. 621.

86. Nordic Nutrition Recommendations 2012: Integrating nutrition and physical activity. 5th ed. Copenhagen: Nordic Nutrition Recommendations 2012; 2014 [cited 2017-11-15]. 627 p (Nord). Available from: http://www.norden.org/en/theme/former-

themes/themes-2016/nordic-nutrition-recommendation/nordic-nutrition-recommendations-2012 p. 622.

87. Nordic Nutrition Recommendations 2012: Integrating nutrition and physical activity. 5th ed. Copenhagen: Nordic Nutrition Recommendations 2012; 2014 [cited 2017-11-15]. 627 p (Nord). Available from: http://www.norden.org/en/theme/former-themes/themes-2016/nordic-nutrition-recommendation/nordic-nutrition-recommendations-2012 p. 623.

88. Nordic Nutrition Recommendations 2012: Integrating nutrition and physical activity. 5th ed. Copenhagen: Nordic Nutrition Recommendations 2012; 2014 [cited 2017-11-16]. 627 p (Nord). Available from: http://www.norden.org/en/theme/former-themes/themes-2016/nordic-nutrition-recommendation/nordic-nutrition-recommendations-2012 p. 336.

89. Witthöft C. Fettlösliga vitaminer [PowerPoint presentation on the Internet]. Kalmar: Linnéuniversitetet; 2016. [cited 26 June 2017]. Available from: https://mymoodle.lnu.se/pluginfile.php/1384387/ mod_resource/content/1/Fettlösliga%20vitaminer %2020160405%20sv.pdf.

90. Nordic Nutrition Recommendations 2012: Integrating nutrition and physical activity. 5th ed. Copenhagen: Nordic Nutrition Recommendations 2012; 2014 [cited 2017-11-16]. 627 p (Nord). Available from: http://www.norden.org/en/theme/former-themes/themes-2016/nordic-nutrition-recommendation/nordic-nutrition-recommendations-2012 p. 337.

91. Nordic Nutrition Recommendations 2012: Integrating nutrition and physical activity. 5th ed. Copenhagen: Nordic Nutrition Recommendations 2012; 2014 [cited 2017-11-16]. 627 p (Nord). Available from: http://www.norden.org/en/theme/former-

themes/themes-2016/nordic-nutrition-recommendation/nordic-nutrition-recommendations-2012 p. 338.

92. Nordic Nutrition Recommendations 2012: Integrating nutrition and physical activity. 5th ed. Copenhagen: Nordic Nutrition Recommendations 2012; 2014 [cited 2017-11-16]. 627 p (Nord). Available from: http://www.norden.org/en/theme/former-themes/themes-2016/nordic-nutrition-recommendation/nordic-nutrition-recommendations-2012 p. 335.

93. Nordic Nutrition Recommendations 2012: Integrating nutrition and physical activity. 5th ed. Copenhagen: Nordic Nutrition Recommendations 2012; 2014 [cited 2017-11-16]. 627 p (Nord). Available from: http://www.norden.org/en/theme/former-themes/themes-2016/nordic-nutrition-recommendation/nordic-nutrition-recommendations-2012 p. 349.

94. Nordic Nutrition Recommendations 2012: Integrating nutrition and physical activity. 5th ed. Copenhagen: Nordic Nutrition Recommendations 2012; 2014 [cited 2017-11-16]. 627 p (Nord). Available from: http://www.norden.org/en/theme/former-themes/themes-2016/nordic-nutrition-recommendation/nordic-nutrition-recommendations-2012 p. 353.

95. Nordic Nutrition Recommendations 2012: Integrating nutrition and physical activity. 5th ed. Copenhagen: Nordic Nutrition Recommendations 2012; 2014 [cited 2017-11-16]. 627 p (Nord). Available from: http://www.norden.org/en/theme/former-themes/themes-2016/nordic-nutrition-recommendation/nordic-nutrition-recommendations-2012 p. 356.

96. Nordic Nutrition Recommendations 2012: Integrating nutrition and physical activity. 5th ed. Copenhagen: Nordic Nutrition Recommendations 2012; 2014 [cited 2017-11-16]. 627 p (Nord).

Available from:

http://www.norden.org/en/theme/former-themes/themes-2016/nordic-nutrition-recommendation/nordic-nutrition-recommendations-2012 p. 371.

97. Nordic Nutrition Recommendations 2012: Integrating nutrition and physical activity. 5th ed. Copenhagen: Nordic Nutrition Recommendations 2012; 2014 [cited 2017-11-16]. 627 p (Nord). Available from:

http://www.norden.org/en/theme/former-themes/themes-2016/nordic-nutrition-recommendation/nordic-nutrition-recommendations-2012 p. 352.

98. Nordic Nutrition Recommendations 2012: Integrating nutrition and physical activity. 5th ed. Copenhagen: Nordic Nutrition Recommendations 2012; 2014 [cited 2017-11-17]. 627 p (Nord). Available from:

http://www.norden.org/en/theme/former-themes/themes-2016/nordic-nutrition-

recommendation/nordic-nutrition-
recommendations-2012 p. 386.

99. Nordic Nutrition Recommendations 2012:
Integrating nutrition and physical activity. 5th ed.
Copenhagen: Nordic Nutrition Recommendations
2012; 2014 [cited 2017-11-17]. 627 p (Nord).
Available from:
http://www.norden.org/en/theme/former-
themes/themes-2016/nordic-nutrition-
recommendation/nordic-nutrition-
recommendations-2012 p. 387.

100. Nordic Nutrition Recommendations 2012:
Integrating nutrition and physical activity. 5th ed.
Copenhagen: Nordic Nutrition Recommendations
2012; 2014 [cited 2017-11-17]. 627 p (Nord).
Available from:
http://www.norden.org/en/theme/former-
themes/themes-2016/nordic-nutrition-
recommendation/nordic-nutrition-
recommendations-2012 p. 388.

101. Nordic Nutrition Recommendations 2012:
Integrating nutrition and physical activity. 5th ed.

Copenhagen: Nordic Nutrition Recommendations
2012; 2014 [cited 2017-11-17]. 627 p (Nord).
Available from:
http://www.norden.org/en/theme/former-
themes/themes-2016/nordic-nutrition-
recommendation/nordic-nutrition-
recommendations-2012 p. 385.

102.   Nordic Nutrition Recommendations 2012:
Integrating nutrition and physical activity. 5th ed.
Copenhagen: Nordic Nutrition Recommendations
2012; 2014 [cited 2017-11-17]. 627 p (Nord).
Available from:
http://www.norden.org/en/theme/former-
themes/themes-2016/nordic-nutrition-
recommendation/nordic-nutrition-
recommendations-2012 p. 399.

103.   Nordic Nutrition Recommendations 2012:
Integrating nutrition and physical activity. 5th ed.
Copenhagen: Nordic Nutrition Recommendations
2012; 2014 [cited 2017-11-17]. 627 p (Nord).
Available from:
http://www.norden.org/en/theme/former-

themes/themes-2016/nordic-nutrition-
recommendation/nordic-nutrition-
recommendations-2012 p. 400.

104.	Nordic Nutrition Recommendations 2012:
Integrating nutrition and physical activity. 5th ed.
Copenhagen: Nordic Nutrition Recommendations
2012; 2014 [cited 2017-11-17]. 627 p (Nord).
Available from:
http://www.norden.org/en/theme/former-
themes/themes-2016/nordic-nutrition-
recommendation/nordic-nutrition-
recommendations-2012 p. 402.

105.	Nordic Nutrition Recommendations 2012:
Integrating nutrition and physical activity. 5th ed.
Copenhagen: Nordic Nutrition Recommendations
2012; 2014 [cited 2017-11-18]. 627 p (Nord).
Available from:
http://www.norden.org/en/theme/former-
themes/themes-2016/nordic-nutrition-
recommendation/nordic-nutrition-
recommendations-2012 p. 465.

106. Nordic Nutrition Recommendations 2012: Integrating nutrition and physical activity. 5th ed. Copenhagen: Nordic Nutrition Recommendations 2012; 2014 [cited 2017-11-18]. 627 p (Nord). Available from: http://www.norden.org/en/theme/former-themes/themes-2016/nordic-nutrition-recommendation/nordic-nutrition-recommendations-2012 p. 466.

107. Nordic Nutrition Recommendations 2012: Integrating nutrition and physical activity. 5th ed. Copenhagen: Nordic Nutrition Recommendations 2012; 2014 [cited 2017-11-18]. 627 p (Nord). Available from: http://www.norden.org/en/theme/former-themes/themes-2016/nordic-nutrition-recommendation/nordic-nutrition-recommendations-2012 p. 467.

108. Witthöft C. The water-soluble vitamins [PowerPoint presentation on the Internet]. Kalmar: Linnéuniversitetet; 2016. [cited 26 June 2017]. Available from:

https://mymoodle.lnu.se/pluginfile.php/1385070/mod_resource/content/1/vattenl%20vitaminer%201%202016.pdf.

109.   Nordic Nutrition Recommendations 2012: Integrating nutrition and physical activity. 5th ed. Copenhagen: Nordic Nutrition Recommendations 2012; 2014 [cited 2017-11-18]. 627 p (Nord). Available from: http://www.norden.org/en/theme/former-themes/themes-2016/nordic-nutrition-recommendation/nordic-nutrition-recommendations-2012 p. 469.

110.   Nordic Nutrition Recommendations 2012: Integrating nutrition and physical activity. 5th ed. Copenhagen: Nordic Nutrition Recommendations 2012; 2014 [cited 2017-11-18]. 627 p (Nord). Available from: http://www.norden.org/en/theme/former-themes/themes-2016/nordic-nutrition-recommendation/nordic-nutrition-recommendations-2012 p. 407.

111.	Nordic Nutrition Recommendations 2012: Integrating nutrition and physical activity. 5th ed. Copenhagen: Nordic Nutrition Recommendations 2012; 2014 [cited 2017-11-18]. 627 p (Nord). Available from: http://www.norden.org/en/theme/former-themes/themes-2016/nordic-nutrition-recommendation/nordic-nutrition-recommendations-2012 p. 408.

112.	Nordic Nutrition Recommendations 2012: Integrating nutrition and physical activity. 5th ed. Copenhagen: Nordic Nutrition Recommendations 2012; 2014 [cited 2017-11-19]. 627 p (Nord). Available from: http://www.norden.org/en/theme/former-themes/themes-2016/nordic-nutrition-recommendation/nordic-nutrition-recommendations-2012 p. 413.

113.	Nordic Nutrition Recommendations 2012: Integrating nutrition and physical activity. 5th ed. Copenhagen: Nordic Nutrition Recommendations 2012; 2014 [cited 2017-11-19]. 627 p (Nord).

Available from:

http://www.norden.org/en/theme/former-
themes/themes-2016/nordic-nutrition-
recommendation/nordic-nutrition-
recommendations-2012 p. 414.

114.   Nordic Nutrition Recommendations 2012:
Integrating nutrition and physical activity. 5th ed.
Copenhagen: Nordic Nutrition Recommendations
2012; 2014 [cited 2017-11-19]. 627 p (Nord).
Available from:
http://www.norden.org/en/theme/former-
themes/themes-2016/nordic-nutrition-
recommendation/nordic-nutrition-
recommendations-2012 p. 419.

115.   Nordic Nutrition Recommendations 2012:
Integrating nutrition and physical activity. 5th ed.
Copenhagen: Nordic Nutrition Recommendations
2012; 2014 [cited 2017-11-19]. 627 p (Nord).
Available from:
http://www.norden.org/en/theme/former-
themes/themes-2016/nordic-nutrition-

recommendation/nordic-nutrition-recommendations-2012 p. 420.

116.   Nordic Nutrition Recommendations 2012: Integrating nutrition and physical activity. 5th ed. Copenhagen: Nordic Nutrition Recommendations 2012; 2014 [cited 2017-11-19]. 627 p (Nord). Available from: http://www.norden.org/en/theme/former-themes/themes-2016/nordic-nutrition-recommendation/nordic-nutrition-recommendations-2012 p. 421.

117.   Nordic Nutrition Recommendations 2012: Integrating nutrition and physical activity. 5th ed. Copenhagen: Nordic Nutrition Recommendations 2012; 2014 [cited 2017-11-19]. 627 p (Nord). Available from: http://www.norden.org/en/theme/former-themes/themes-2016/nordic-nutrition-recommendation/nordic-nutrition-recommendations-2012 p. 463.

118.   Nordic Nutrition Recommendations 2012: Integrating nutrition and physical activity. 5th ed.

Copenhagen: Nordic Nutrition Recommendations 2012; 2014 [cited 2017-11-19]. 627 p (Nord). Available from: http://www.norden.org/en/theme/former-themes/themes-2016/nordic-nutrition-recommendation/nordic-nutrition-recommendations-2012 p. 464.

119. Nordic Nutrition Recommendations 2012: Integrating nutrition and physical activity. 5th ed. Copenhagen: Nordic Nutrition Recommendations 2012; 2014 [cited 2017-11-20]. 627 p (Nord). Available from: http://www.norden.org/en/theme/former-themes/themes-2016/nordic-nutrition-recommendation/nordic-nutrition-recommendations-2012 p. 423.

120. Nordic Nutrition Recommendations 2012: Integrating nutrition and physical activity. 5th ed. Copenhagen: Nordic Nutrition Recommendations 2012; 2014 [cited 2017-11-20]. 627 p (Nord). Available from: http://www.norden.org/en/theme/former-

themes/themes-2016/nordic-nutrition-recommendation/nordic-nutrition-recommendations-2012 p. 424.

121.   Nordic Nutrition Recommendations 2012: Integrating nutrition and physical activity. 5th ed. Copenhagen: Nordic Nutrition Recommendations 2012; 2014 [cited 2017-11-20]. 627 p (Nord). Available from: http://www.norden.org/en/theme/former-themes/themes-2016/nordic-nutrition-recommendation/nordic-nutrition-recommendations-2012 p. 425.

122.   Nordic Nutrition Recommendations 2012: Integrating nutrition and physical activity. 5th ed. Copenhagen: Nordic Nutrition Recommendations 2012; 2014 [cited 2017-11-20]. 627 p (Nord). Available from: http://www.norden.org/en/theme/former-themes/themes-2016/nordic-nutrition-recommendation/nordic-nutrition-recommendations-2012 p. 430.

123.   Nordic Nutrition Recommendations 2012: Integrating nutrition and physical activity. 5th ed. Copenhagen: Nordic Nutrition Recommendations 2012; 2014 [cited 2017-11-20]. 627 p (Nord). Available from: http://www.norden.org/en/theme/former-themes/themes-2016/nordic-nutrition-recommendation/nordic-nutrition-recommendations-2012 p. 459.

124.   Nordic Nutrition Recommendations 2012: Integrating nutrition and physical activity. 5th ed. Copenhagen: Nordic Nutrition Recommendations 2012; 2014 [cited 2017-11-20]. 627 p (Nord). Available from: http://www.norden.org/en/theme/former-themes/themes-2016/nordic-nutrition-recommendation/nordic-nutrition-recommendations-2012 p. 460.

125.   Nordic Nutrition Recommendations 2012: Integrating nutrition and physical activity. 5th ed. Copenhagen: Nordic Nutrition Recommendations 2012; 2014 [cited 2017-11-20]. 627 p (Nord).

Available from:

http://www.norden.org/en/theme/former-themes/themes-2016/nordic-nutrition-recommendation/nordic-nutrition-recommendations-2012 p. 435.

126.   Nordic Nutrition Recommendations 2012: Integrating nutrition and physical activity. 5th ed. Copenhagen: Nordic Nutrition Recommendations 2012; 2014 [cited 2017-11-20]. 627 p (Nord). Available from: http://www.norden.org/en/theme/former-themes/themes-2016/nordic-nutrition-recommendation/nordic-nutrition-recommendations-2012 p. 436.

127.   Nordic Nutrition Recommendations 2012: Integrating nutrition and physical activity. 5th ed. Copenhagen: Nordic Nutrition Recommendations 2012; 2014 [cited 2017-11-20]. 627 p (Nord). Available from: http://www.norden.org/en/theme/former-themes/themes-2016/nordic-nutrition-

recommendation/nordic-nutrition-recommendations-2012 p. 437.

128.   Nordic Nutrition Recommendations 2012: Integrating nutrition and physical activity. 5th ed. Copenhagen: Nordic Nutrition Recommendations 2012; 2014 [cited 2017-11-20]. 627 p (Nord). Available from: http://www.norden.org/en/theme/former-themes/themes-2016/nordic-nutrition-recommendation/nordic-nutrition-recommendations-2012 p. 444.

129.   Nordic Nutrition Recommendations 2012: Integrating nutrition and physical activity. 5th ed. Copenhagen: Nordic Nutrition Recommendations 2012; 2014 [cited 2017-11-21]. 627 p (Nord). Available from: http://www.norden.org/en/theme/former-themes/themes-2016/nordic-nutrition-recommendation/nordic-nutrition-recommendations-2012 p. 449.

130.   Nordic Nutrition Recommendations 2012: Integrating nutrition and physical activity. 5th ed.

Copenhagen: Nordic Nutrition Recommendations 2012; 2014 [cited 2017-11-21]. 627 p (Nord). Available from: http://www.norden.org/en/theme/former-themes/themes-2016/nordic-nutrition-recommendation/nordic-nutrition-recommendations-2012 p. 450.

131.   Nordic Nutrition Recommendations 2012: Integrating nutrition and physical activity. 5th ed. Copenhagen: Nordic Nutrition Recommendations 2012; 2014 [cited 2017-11-21]. 627 p (Nord). Available from: http://www.norden.org/en/theme/former-themes/themes-2016/nordic-nutrition-recommendation/nordic-nutrition-recommendations-2012 p. 451.

132.   Nordic Nutrition Recommendations 2012: Integrating nutrition and physical activity. 5th ed. Copenhagen: Nordic Nutrition Recommendations 2012; 2014 [cited 2017-11-21]. 627 p (Nord). Available from: http://www.norden.org/en/theme/former-

themes/themes-2016/nordic-nutrition-recommendation/nordic-nutrition-recommendations-2012 p. 455.

133. Blücher A. Kolhydrater [PowerPoint presentation on the Internet]. Kalmar: Linnéuniversitetet; 2016. [cited 27 June 2017]. Available from: https://mymoodle.lnu.se/pluginfile.php/1318343/mod_resource/content/4/Anna_B/Kolhydrat_16_nutrition%20och%20näringslära-3.pdf.

134. Nordic Nutrition Recommendations 2012: Integrating nutrition and physical activity. 5th ed. Copenhagen: Nordic Nutrition Recommendations 2012; 2014 [cited 2017-11-23]. 627 p (Nord). Available from: http://www.norden.org/en/theme/former-themes/themes-2016/nordic-nutrition-recommendation/nordic-nutrition-recommendations-2012 p. 250.

135. Nordic Nutrition Recommendations 2012: Integrating nutrition and physical activity. 5th ed. Copenhagen: Nordic Nutrition Recommendations

2012; 2014 [cited 2017-11-23]. 627 p (Nord).
Available from:
http://www.norden.org/en/theme/former-themes/themes-2016/nordic-nutrition-recommendation/nordic-nutrition-recommendations-2012 p. 251.

136.   Nordic Nutrition Recommendations 2012: Integrating nutrition and physical activity. 5th ed. Copenhagen: Nordic Nutrition Recommendations 2012; 2014 [cited 2017-11-23]. 627 p (Nord). Available from:
http://www.norden.org/en/theme/former-themes/themes-2016/nordic-nutrition-recommendation/nordic-nutrition-recommendations-2012 p. 254.

137.   Nordic Nutrition Recommendations 2012: Integrating nutrition and physical activity. 5th ed. Copenhagen: Nordic Nutrition Recommendations 2012; 2014 [cited 2017-11-23]. 627 p (Nord). Available from:
http://www.norden.org/en/theme/former-themes/themes-2016/nordic-nutrition-

recommendation/nordic-nutrition-recommendations-2012 p. 255.

138.   Nordic Nutrition Recommendations 2012: Integrating nutrition and physical activity. 5th ed. Copenhagen: Nordic Nutrition Recommendations 2012; 2014 [cited 2017-11-23]. 627 p (Nord). Available from: http://www.norden.org/en/theme/former-themes/themes-2016/nordic-nutrition-recommendation/nordic-nutrition-recommendations-2012 p. 257.

139.   Nordic Nutrition Recommendations 2012: Integrating nutrition and physical activity. 5th ed. Copenhagen: Nordic Nutrition Recommendations 2012; 2014 [cited 2017-11-23]. 627 p (Nord). Available from: http://www.norden.org/en/theme/former-themes/themes-2016/nordic-nutrition-recommendation/nordic-nutrition-recommendations-2012 p. 249.

140.   Nordic Nutrition Recommendations 2012: Integrating nutrition and physical activity. 5th ed.

Copenhagen: Nordic Nutrition Recommendations
2012; 2014 [cited 2017-11-23]. 627 p (Nord).
Available from:
http://www.norden.org/en/theme/former-
themes/themes-2016/nordic-nutrition-
recommendation/nordic-nutrition-
recommendations-2012 p. 26.

141.   Nordic Nutrition Recommendations 2012:
Integrating nutrition and physical activity. 5th ed.
Copenhagen: Nordic Nutrition Recommendations
2012; 2014 [cited 2017-11-23]. 627 p (Nord).
Available from:
http://www.norden.org/en/theme/former-
themes/themes-2016/nordic-nutrition-
recommendation/nordic-nutrition-
recommendations-2012 p. 27.

142.   Nordic Nutrition Recommendations 2012:
Integrating nutrition and physical activity. 5th ed.
Copenhagen: Nordic Nutrition Recommendations
2012; 2014 [cited 2017-11-23]. 627 p (Nord).
Available from:
http://www.norden.org/en/theme/former-

themes/themes-2016/nordic-nutrition-
recommendation/nordic-nutrition-
recommendations-2012 p. 261.

143.	Nordic Nutrition Recommendations 2012:
Integrating nutrition and physical activity. 5th ed.
Copenhagen: Nordic Nutrition Recommendations
2012; 2014 [cited 2017-11-23]. 627 p (Nord).
Available from:
http://www.norden.org/en/theme/former-
themes/themes-2016/nordic-nutrition-
recommendation/nordic-nutrition-
recommendations-2012 p. 262.

144.	Nordic Nutrition Recommendations 2012:
Integrating nutrition and physical activity. 5th ed.
Copenhagen: Nordic Nutrition Recommendations
2012; 2014 [cited 2017-11-23]. 627 p (Nord).
Available from:
http://www.norden.org/en/theme/former-
themes/themes-2016/nordic-nutrition-
recommendation/nordic-nutrition-
recommendations-2012 p. 269.

145. Nordic Nutrition Recommendations 2012: Integrating nutrition and physical activity. 5th ed. Copenhagen: Nordic Nutrition Recommendations 2012; 2014 [cited 2017-11-23]. 627 p (Nord). Available from: http://www.norden.org/en/theme/former-themes/themes-2016/nordic-nutrition-recommendation/nordic-nutrition-recommendations-2012 p. 270.

146. Nordic Nutrition Recommendations 2012: Integrating nutrition and physical activity. 5th ed. Copenhagen: Nordic Nutrition Recommendations 2012; 2014 [cited 2017-11-23]. 627 p (Nord). Available from: http://www.norden.org/en/theme/former-themes/themes-2016/nordic-nutrition-recommendation/nordic-nutrition-recommendations-2012 p. 272.

147. Edman K. Proteiner [PowerPoint presentation on the Internet]. Kalmar: Linnéuniversitetet; 2016. [cited 28 June 2017]. Available from:

https://mymoodle.lnu.se/course/view.php?id=192
66.

148. Nordic Nutrition Recommendations 2012:
Integrating nutrition and physical activity. 5th ed.
Copenhagen: Nordic Nutrition Recommendations
2012; 2014 [cited 2017-11-24]. 627 p (Nord).
Available from:
http://www.norden.org/en/theme/former-
themes/themes-2016/nordic-nutrition-
recommendation/nordic-nutrition-
recommendations-2012 p. 281.

149. Nordic Nutrition Recommendations 2012:
Integrating nutrition and physical activity. 5th ed.
Copenhagen: Nordic Nutrition Recommendations
2012; 2014 [cited 2017-11-24]. 627 p (Nord).
Available from:
http://www.norden.org/en/theme/former-
themes/themes-2016/nordic-nutrition-
recommendation/nordic-nutrition-
recommendations-2012 p. 291.

150. Nordic Nutrition Recommendations 2012:
Integrating nutrition and physical activity. 5th ed.

Copenhagen: Nordic Nutrition Recommendations 2012; 2014 [cited 2017-11-24]. 627 p (Nord). Available from: http://www.norden.org/en/theme/former-themes/themes-2016/nordic-nutrition-recommendation/nordic-nutrition-recommendations-2012 p. 292.

151.   Nordic Nutrition Recommendations 2012: Integrating nutrition and physical activity. 5th ed. Copenhagen: Nordic Nutrition Recommendations 2012; 2014 [cited 2017-11-24]. 627 p (Nord). Available from: http://www.norden.org/en/theme/former-themes/themes-2016/nordic-nutrition-recommendation/nordic-nutrition-recommendations-2012 p. 295.

152.   Nordic Nutrition Recommendations 2012: Integrating nutrition and physical activity. 5th ed. Copenhagen: Nordic Nutrition Recommendations 2012; 2014 [cited 2017-11-24]. 627 p (Nord). Available from: http://www.norden.org/en/theme/former-

themes/themes-2016/nordic-nutrition-recommendation/nordic-nutrition-recommendations-2012 p. 296.

153.   Persson AA. Fettmetabolism [PowerPoint presentation on the Internet]. Kalmar: Linnéuniversitetet; 2016. [cited June 29 2017]. Available from: https://mymoodle.lnu.se/mod/folder/view.php?id=952244.

154.   Nordic Nutrition Recommendations 2012: Integrating nutrition and physical activity. 5th ed. Copenhagen: Nordic Nutrition Recommendations 2012; 2014 [cited 2017-11-25]. 627 p (Nord). Available from: http://www.norden.org/en/theme/former-themes/themes-2016/nordic-nutrition-recommendation/nordic-nutrition-recommendations-2012 p. 217.

155.   Nordic Nutrition Recommendations 2012: Integrating nutrition and physical activity. 5th ed. Copenhagen: Nordic Nutrition Recommendations

2012; 2014 [cited 2017-11-25]. 627 p (Nord).
Available from:
http://www.norden.org/en/theme/former-themes/themes-2016/nordic-nutrition-recommendation/nordic-nutrition-recommendations-2012 p. 25.

156.   Nordic Nutrition Recommendations 2012:
Integrating nutrition and physical activity. 5th ed.
Copenhagen: Nordic Nutrition Recommendations
2012; 2014 [cited 2017-11-25]. 627 p (Nord).
Available from:
http://www.norden.org/en/theme/former-themes/themes-2016/nordic-nutrition-recommendation/nordic-nutrition-recommendations-2012 p. 26.

157.   Nordic Nutrition Recommendations 2012:
Integrating nutrition and physical activity. 5th ed.
Copenhagen: Nordic Nutrition Recommendations
2012; 2014 [cited 2017-11-25]. 627 p (Nord).
Available from:
http://www.norden.org/en/theme/former-themes/themes-2016/nordic-nutrition-

recommendation/nordic-nutrition-
recommendations-2012 p. 230.

158.   Centers for Disease Control and Prevention.
Finding a Balance [Internet]. USA: Centers for
Disease Control and Prevention; 2016 [updated
date 2016-11-16; cited 2017 August 29].
Available from:
https://www.cdc.gov/healthyweight/calories/index
.html.

159.   Eneroth, H Björck, L Konde, ÅB. Bra
livsmedelsval baserat på nordiska
näringsrekommendationer 2012. Uppsala:
Livsmedelsverket; 2014 [read 2017-12-02].
Available from:
https://mymoodle.lnu.se/pluginfile.php/1318328/
mod_resource/content/1/2014_livsmedelsverket_
19_bra_livsmedelsval.pdf.

160.   Paulún F. 50 genvägar till fettförbränning.
Falun: ScandBook AB; 2014. P. 113

161.   Reygaert WC. An update on the health
benefits of green tea. Beverages. 2017;3(1):6

162. Lee KW, Lee HJ, Lee CY. Antioxidant activity of black tea vs. green tea. J Nutr. 2002 Apr;132(4):785.

163. Paulún F. 50 genvägar till fettförbränning. Falun: ScandBook AB; 2014. P. 102

164. Paulún F. 50 genvägar till fettförbränning. Falun: ScandBook AB; 2014. P. 103

165. Bae JH, Park JH, Im SS, Song DK. Coffee and health. Integr Med Res. 2014 Dec;3(4):189-191.

166. Paulún F. 50 genvägar till fettförbränning. Falun: ScandBook AB; 2014. P. 108

167. Paulún F. 50 genvägar till fettförbränning. Falun: ScandBook AB; 2014. P. 107

168. Nordic Nutrition Recommendations 2012: Integrating nutrition and physical activity. 5th ed. Copenhagen: Nordic Nutrition Recommendations 2012; 2014 [cited 2017-11-26]. 627 p (Nord). Available from: http://www.norden.org/en/theme/former-themes/themes-2016/nordic-nutrition-

recommendation/nordic-nutrition-recommendations-2012 p. 311

169. Nordic Nutrition Recommendations 2012: Integrating nutrition and physical activity. 5th ed. Copenhagen: Nordic Nutrition Recommendations 2012; 2014 [cited 2017-11-26]. 627 p (Nord). Available from: http://www.norden.org/en/theme/former-themes/themes-2016/nordic-nutrition-recommendation/nordic-nutrition-recommendations-2012 p. 312.

170. Paulún F. 50 genvägar till fettförbränning. Falun: ScandBook AB; 2014. P. 116

171. Paulún F. 50 genvägar till fettförbränning. Falun: ScandBook AB; 2014. P. 117

172. Paulún F. 50 genvägar till fettförbränning. Falun: ScandBook AB; 2014. P. 118

173. Paulún F. 50 genvägar till fettförbränning. Falun: ScandBook AB; 2014. P. 120

174. Nordic Nutrition Recommendations 2012: Integrating nutrition and physical activity. 5th ed. Copenhagen: Nordic Nutrition Recommendations

2012; 2014 [cited 2017-11-26]. 627 p (Nord).
Available from:
http://www.norden.org/en/theme/former-themes/themes-2016/nordic-nutrition-recommendation/nordic-nutrition-recommendations-2012 p. 318.

175.   Nordic Nutrition Recommendations 2012:
Integrating nutrition and physical activity. 5th ed.
Copenhagen: Nordic Nutrition Recommendations
2012; 2014 [cited 2017-11-26]. 627 p (Nord).
Available from:
http://www.norden.org/en/theme/former-themes/themes-2016/nordic-nutrition-recommendation/nordic-nutrition-recommendations-2012 p. 319.

176.   Strasser B, Schobergsberger W. Evidence
for resistance training as a treatment therapy in
obesity. J Obes. 2011;2011.

177.   Hills AP, Schultz SP, Soares MJ, Byrne
NM, Hunter GR, King NA, et al. Resistance
training for obese, type 2 diabetic adults: a review

of the evidence. Obes Rev. 2010 Oct;11(10):740-9.

178.   Lopes WA, Leite N, da Silva LR, Brunelli DT, Gáspari AF, Radominski RB, et al. Effects of 12 weeks of combined training without caloric restriction on inflammatory markers in overweight girls. J Sports Sci. 2016 Oct;34(20):1902-12.

179.   Ho SS, Dhaliwal SS, Hills AP, Pal S. The effect of 12 weeks of aerobic, resistance or combination exercise training on cardiovascular risk factors in the overweight and obese in a randomized trial. BMC Public Health. 2012 Aug 28;12:704.

180.   AbouAssi H, Slentz CA, Mikus CR, Tanner CJ, Bateman LA, Willis LH, et al. The effects of aerobic, resistance, and combination training on insulin sensitivity and secretion in overweight adults from STRRIDE AT/RT: a randomized trial. J Appl Physiol (1985). 2015 Jun 15;118(12):1474-82.

181.   Wycherley TP, Noakes M, Clifton PM, Cleanthous X, Keogh JB, Brinkworth GD. A High-Protein Diet With Resistance Exercise Training Improves Weight Loss and Body Composition in Overweight and Obese Patients With Type 2 Diabetes. Diabetes Care. 2010 May;33(5):969-76.

182.   Sachleen K, Anu S, Ajit G, Jagmohan S. Effect of submaximal aerobic exercise on obesity. Indian J Physiother Occup Ther. 2013 Apr-Jun;7(2):161-5.

183.   Willis LH, Slentz CA, Bateman LA, Shields AT, Piner LW, Bales CW, et al. Effects of aerobic and/or resistance training on body mass and fat mass in overweight or obese adults. J Appl Physiol (1985). 2012 Dec 15;113(12):1831-7.

184.   Lynch N, Nicklas B, Berman D, Dennis K, Goldberg A. Reductions in visceral fat during weight loss and walking are associated with improvements in VO2max. J Appl Physiol. 2001 Jan;90(1):99-104.

185.   Achten J, Jeukendrup AE. Optimizing fat oxidation through exercise and diet. Nutrition. 2004 Jul-Aug;20(7-8):716-27.

186.   Van Proeyen K, Szlufcik K, Nielens H, Ramaekers M, Hespel P. Beneficial metabolic adaptations due to endurance exercise training in the fasted state. J Appl Physiol (1985). 2011 Jan;110(1):236-45.

187.   Van Proeyen K, Szlufcik K, Nielens H, Pelgrim K, Deldicque L, Hesselink M, et al. Training in the fasted state improves glucose tolerance during fat-rich diet. J Physiol. 2010 Nov 1;588(Pt 21):4289-302.

188.   De Bock K, Ricther EA, Russell AP, Eijnde BO, Derave W, Ramaekers M, et al. Exercise in the fasted state facilitates fibre type-specific intramyocellular lipid breakdown and stimulates glycogen resynthesis in humans. J Physiol. 2005 Apr 15;564(Pt 2):649-60.

189.   Calculator: calorie calculator: calculator; 2008 – 2018 [cited 2018 January 23]. Available

from: http://www.calculator.net/calorie-calculator.html.

Appendix

Here I will describe how to perform the exercises in a correct way. Since, no gym in my home town allowed to record videos in gyms I couldn't record the videos for you. But if you don't understand any of the exercises below, I would recommend you to watch YouTube videos on how to perform the exercises, and if you don't understand how to do the exercises when you have watched YouTube videos, then I would recommend you to ask a personal trainer at a gym or you can ask me on e-mail and I will describe the parts you don't understand.

Bench Press (Machine)

When you perform the bench press on a machine, there are some important things to remember. First you want to adjust the seat so the bottom chest is in the height with the handles. Then you want to adjust the handles so that you start the movement in a 90-degree angle with your elbows. You will also make sure that your legs are in a 90-degree angle. Now, pick a weight that you can do for at least 8 reps and max 12 reps in a controlled way, it should be very low when you perform the exercise for the first time. The reason why you pick a low weight is because you don't want to get injured. When you have picked a weight, you will put your head against the pad so that you maintain a neutral spine. It's very important that you don't bend your wrists, because the wrists will stay straight during the movement. When you push the weight forward, you will breathe out and when you release the pressure to the starting position, you will breathe in. Go back to the starting position which is a 90-degree angle with your elbows and then push again for 8 – 12 reps. This is how you do the bench press on a machine. If you don't understand how to do the exercise, there are always people at gyms that will help you.

Lat Pull Downs (Machine)

When you perform the lat pull down on a machine, there are some important things to remember. First, you want to adjust the pads in front of the seat so that they are on top of your quadriceps, so you stay in the correct position during the whole movement. Pick a weight that you can do for at least 8 reps and max 12 reps in a controlled way, it should be very low when you perform the exercise for the first time. Now, you want to grab the handles above you and keep your wrists straight during the movement, keep your head up so that you maintain a neutral spine, sit down and lock your legs under the pad in front of the seat, so that you sit in a position that feels safe. Now, you want to start the movement, pull the handles down so that your hands are just over shoulders and just below your chin, then go back up over your head until your elbows are slightly bent at the top movement, this will keep your muscles activated during the entire movement. If you would go back until your elbows are straight, then your muscles won't be activated, so try to keep a slightly bend of your elbows at the top position. You will breathe out when you pull the handles down and you will breathe in when you go back up during the movement. You will always breathe out when you perform the heavy part of the movement. Never let the handles go below your shoulders, because then you will activate other muscles and the risk for injury increases. This is how you do the lat pull down on a machine. If you don't understand how to do the exercise, there are always people at gyms that will help you.

Shoulder Press (Machine)

When you perform the shoulder press on a machine, there are some important things to remember. First, you want to pick a weight that you can do for at least 8 reps and max 12 reps in a controlled way, it should be very low when you perform the exercise for the first time. Then you will adjust the seat so that your elbows are in an almost 90-degree angle in the start of the movement. Make sure that your elbows are in line with your hips and pointed forward during the movement, because this will increase the stimulus in the muscles on the back of your shoulder. Grab the handles and keep your wrists straight and maintain a neutral spine by putting your head against the head pad. Push the handles to the starting position (an almost 90-degree angle with your elbows), then, push the weight up until your elbows are slightly bent at the top of the movement, go then back down to 90-degrees with your elbows. Breathe out on the way up and breathe in on the way down. Do this for 8 – 12 reps. This is how you do the shoulder press on a machine. If you don't understand how to do the exercise, there are always people at gyms that will help you.

Lateral Raises (Machine)

When you perform the lateral raises on a machine, there are some important things to remember. First, you want to pick a weight that you can do for at least 8 reps and max 12 reps in a controlled way, it should be very low when you perform the exercise for the first time. Then you want to adjust the seat so that your arms are in line with the pads while you grip the handles. Keep your elbows beside the ribs, chest high and your head up. Then, lift through the elbow joint until the arms are in the height with the shoulders. At the top position of the movement, your hands, elbows and shoulder should all be in line with each other. Breathe out on the way up and breathe in on the way down. You will keep the elbows in touch with the pads during the entire movement. This is how you do the lateral raises on a machine. If you don't understand how to do the exercise, there are always people at gyms that will help you.

Biceps Curls (Machine)

When you perform the biceps curls on a machine, there are some important things to remember. First, you want to adjust the seat so that you sit comfortable on the seat. Then you want to pick a weight that you can do for at least 8 reps and max 12 reps in a controlled way, it should be very low when you perform the exercise for the first time. Now, grab the handles and make sure that your palms of the hand are faced up during the entire movement. Your forearms will get more stimulus when your palms are faced up. Position your elbows so that they are in line with the pivot point of the machine. Sit up straight, keep your head up, maintain a neutral spine, keep your wrists straight. Now, you will start the movement, bring the handles up so that the elbows are in a little more than 90-degree angle. Go down until your elbows are slightly bent. Breathe out on the way up and breathe in on the way down. This is how you do the biceps curls on a machine. If you don't understand how to do the exercise, there are always people at gyms that will help you.

Triceps Extensions (Machine)

When you perform the triceps extension on a machine, there are some important things to remember. First, you want to pick a weight that you can do for at least 8 reps and max 12 reps in a controlled way, it should be very low when you perform the exercise for the first time. Then, you will adjust the height of the seat and adjust the back seat so that you sit comfortable. Your elbows will be in the line with the pivot point of the machine. Grab the handles and place your arms on the pad. You will make sure that your elbows are in a 90-degree angle and that the handles are in the height of your nose in the starting position. Keep your feet in front of you on the floor. Keep your elbows in line with your shoulder and keep your wrists straight. Breathe out on the way down and breathe in on the way back up. You will go down until the elbows are in a slightly bent angle, not straight, but just a slightly bend, then you will go back up to the starting position (the elbows will be in a 90-degree angle and the handles will be in the height of your nose). This is how you do the triceps extensions on a machine. If you don't understand how to do the exercise, there are always people at gyms that will help you.

Leg Press (Machine)

When you perform the leg press on a machine, there are some important things to remember. First, you want to adjust the back seat so that you sit comfortable. Then you want to adjust how far away from the leg pad that your legs will be. Your legs will be in a 90-degree angle in the starting position. Pick a weight that you can do for at least 8 reps and max 12 reps in a controlled way, it should be very low when you perform the exercise for the first time. Put your head against the head pad so that you maintain a neutral spine. Place the feet on the pad in front of you and make sure that the toes are over your knees. You never want the knees to over your toes because then the pressure will be on your knees, and that is something that we don't want. We want the stimulus in the leg muscles. Grab the handles. Now you will start the movement, push off through your heels, and push forward until your knees are bent at the top position of the movement, then go back to a 90-degree angle. You don't want the weights to touch because then you are not activating your muscles anymore. Breathe out when you push off and breathe in when you go back. This is how you do the leg press on a machine. If you don't understand how to do the exercise, there are always people at gyms that will help you.

Calves Press (Machine)

When you perform the calves press on a machine, there are some important things to remember. You can do this exercise on the leg press machine, it works perfect. Pick a weight that you can do for at least 8 reps and max 12 reps in a controlled way, it should be very low when you perform the exercise for the first time. First, place your feet on the board so that your toes are on the board and your heels down below the bottom where the board ends. Keep your toes straight. Keep your head and back against the pad so you maintain a neutral spine. Push off with your toes and go back with your heels. Your knees will be slightly bent during the entire motion. This is how you do the calves press on a machine. If you don't understand how to do the exercise, there are always people at gyms that will help you.

Sit-Ups (Machine)

When you perform the sit-ups on a machine, there are some important things to remember. First, you want to adjust the height of the seat so that your fist fits in the hole between the back-seat pad and the sit pad. Pick a weight that you can do for at least 8 reps and max 12 reps in a controlled way, it should be very low when you perform the exercise for the first time. Place your feet under the two pads down in front of you on the machine and keep your toes up, lean backwards and keep the shoulders in line with the pad. Keep your head back so that you maintain a neutral spine, grab the handles. Look at something in front of you during the entire movement. Now, you want to start the movement, go down and look at that thing you want to focus on, go back up until you almost hit the starting position, but don't go so far back so you don't activate your muscles anymore. Go back until the weights almost hit each other. Breathe out on the way down and breathe in on the way back. This is how you do the sit-ups on a machine. If you don't understand how to do the exercise, there are always people at gyms that will help you.

Side-to-Sides (Machine)

When you perform the side-to-sides on a machine, there are some important things to remember. First, you want to pick a weight that you can do for at least 8 reps and max 12 reps in a controlled way, it should be very low when you perform the exercise for the first time. Adjust the height of the seat so that your fist fits in the hole between the back-seat pad and the sit pad. Your shoulders will be in line with the back-seat pad. Have a seat on the side with your feet positioned under the leg pads. The edge of the seat will be between your legs. You want to face your oblique (the side of the stomach) as straight as possible forward. Make sure you maintain a neutral spine, look at something in front of you so that your head is up. Breathe out when you go down and breathe in when you come back up. Don't let the weight touch on the way back. When you are finished with one side switch to the other side and do the same movement.

This is how you do the side-to-sides on a machine. If you don't understand how to do the exercise, there are always people at gyms that will help you. This one is a little tricky, but I know you can do it. Watch a YouTube video if you don't understand how you will perform the exercise.

Back Extensions (Machine)

When you perform the back extensions on a machine, there are some important things to remember. First, pick a weight that you can do for at least 8 reps and max 12 reps in a controlled way, it should be very low when you perform the exercise for the first time. The reason why you pick a low weight is because you don't want to get injured. Have a seat and place your feet on the footplate so that you can come in with your back at the lumbar support. Adjust the pad behind you so that you come down to a 90-degree angle. Grip the handles and push your bum back in to the lumbar support again. Keep your head up and chest high during the entire motion. Extend backwards and then go back to your starting position. Don't have a starting position that is deeper than 90-

degrees. This is how you do the back extensions on a machine. If you don't understand how to do the exercise, there are always people at gyms that will help you.